Southwestern
MEDICAL
DICTIONARY

Spanish / *English*
English / *Spanish*

Southwestern
MEDICAL
DICTIONARY

MARGARITA ARTSCHWAGER KAY

with

JOHN D. MEREDITH
WENDY REDLINGER
and
ALICIA QUIROZ RAYMOND

UNIVERSITY OF ARIZONA PRESS
Tucson & London

About the Author . . .

Margarita Artschwager Kay has worked as a public health nurse with Spanish-speakers of the southwestern United States, as well as with patients from Mexico, Central America and Puerto Rico. Her predoctoral and postdoctoral research in the ethnosemantics of health, disease and reproduction led her directly to this book, fusing her knowledge of linguistics, anthropology and health care. As associate professor in the College of Nursing at the University of Arizona, Margarita Kay has taught courses in maternal-newborn nursing and clinical anthropology.

Research for this volume was partially supported by Grant R01 HD07480 from the National Institute of Child Health and Human Development.

Seventh printing 1994

THE UNIVERSITY OF ARIZONA PRESS

ISBN 0-8165-0602-7 cloth
ISBN 0-8165-0529-2 paper
L.C. No. 76-54591

CONTENTS

FOREWORD

Margarita Kay's *Southwestern Medical Dictionary* pulls together all the advantages of four kinds of conventional dictionaries: it is bilingual, technical, regional, and colloquial. Such knowledge usually is not easily accessible to the non-native, since the terms are generally transmitted orally and occur when a particular subject is being discussed in fairly intimate circumstances.

Of the four kinds of dictionaries, the technical bilingual is notable for the sharp focus it gives to specialized terms pertaining to a profession. A dictionary of regionalisms affords a measure of predictability concerning probable as opposed to possible usage. Items collected from actual speech add the dimension of contemporaneousness. This dictionary includes all these qualities.

It contains some 1,200 separate entries in English and more than 1,300 in Spanish. The items are arranged alphabetically with *ch* and *ll* placed conventionally in the Spanish section after *c* and *l*. Included with each definition are part of speech, gender for nouns, Latin name of plants, equivalent medical terminology, a sentence which incorporates the term and a translation of the entire sentence. Special attention is given to expressions with ethnic and colloquial significance. Different kinds of type aid in quick identification (bold face type for the entry, Roman type for the example, and italics for the translation). Data contained in this dictionary were gathered from conversations and interviews held with female informants at a health center in Tucson, Arizona. Many terms were corroborated later in male informants' speech as well. Note-taking and transcriptions were undertaken with the informants' knowledge.

The ever-changing character of spoken language makes imperative the recording of contemporary usage. Margarita Kay and her colleagues have done the medical profession, linguists, historians, and ethnologists a great professional service by compiling terms currently in use by Spanish-speaking people in the Southwest. Because it will serve the important humanitarian end of increasing understanding between medical personnel and patients, the dictionary also stands as a worthy contribution to bilingual studies.

Dolores Brown

INTRODUCTION

In the interest of better communication between patients and health care workers, this book offers words used by Spanish-speaking people on both sides of the Mexico-United States border, with English translations closest to the intended meaning when the concepts are similar. It is unlike other bilingual medical dictionaries that emphasize scientific words which are often cognates, coming from the same classical Greek or Latin. Since the lay person frequently does not understand such words, it makes little difference if they are offered in English or Spanish. This dictionary is also different from the books which translate directions and commands to patients, as its purpose is to help the patient tell his story and the medical practitioner to understand it.

The need for the dictionary became apparent when I was teaching interpreters at a clinic. Here native speakers of Spanish had been used, with little success, to translate the English questions of the health care workers and the Spanish replies of the patients. It was evident that four kinds of translation problems were confounding communication between clients and medical personnel, and these four problems reappeared in the compilation of this dictionary.

The first problem, already suggested, concerns cognitive differences between specialists trained in a specific science and lay people. Because of differing information about what constitutes illness, the basic premises of scientific medicine are not shared. In the absence of shared ideas, simple translation will not work. It is lay terms that are needed, rather than scientific terms in either language.

A second problem occurs when there are different ideas about physiology and pathology, resulting in obstacles to conceptual transfer. Communication about folk diseases is affected by this problem, which, with its related components of herbal treatments and administering curers, is treated as "ethnological" in this dictionary.

A third difficulty arises from insufficient or inaccurate information or inadequate vocabulary. Knowledge of medical language, whether scientific, lay, or folk, reflects personal experience and interest, as well as education. Our informants and their backgrounds were varied, ranging from illegal recent immigrants

to retired *curanderas* (curers) long since em-
igrated from Mexico, second-generation pro-
fessors of nonmedical studies, and third-
generation adolescents who had dropped out
of school. Some of these informants maintained close ties with Mexico; others had
never been there.

Language change, with differential rates for
different individuals, was a fourth problem.
Vocabulary derives from experiences. Despite
the efforts of academicians to keep the
Spanish language pure, medical terminology
continues to reflect both the new technology
and the new "folk medicine" of the various
media, especially radio and television. The
latter in particular affected the medical vocabulary of our youthful informants.

Regional dialect differences have always
affected medical communication. The Spanish
in this dictionary is most accurately called
norteño Spanish, or the Spanish of southern
Arizona and of Sonora, the old Pimería Alta.
Because southern Colorado and northern New
Mexico were isolated from the rest of the
Southwest for long periods of history, some
different words are used in these regions. In
Los Angeles, migration of impoverished
groups from Texas and from central Mexico
has resulted in the selection of some other
concepts and terminology. But because the
differences seem to be fewer than the similar-
ities, we have chosen to call the Spanish in

this book "Southwestern Spanish." Certainly students of Puerto Rican and Cuban-American Spanish will note many more differences.

The lexicon itself is an outgrowth of a glossary which I first prepared for teaching with the encouragement of Demetrio Pacheco. The first version was reworked by Alicia Quíroz Raymond, a native Spanish speaker and a doctoral candidate in Spanish, for teaching a course in medical Spanish. Additional words were collected during interviews for a project titled "The Ethno-semantics of Mexican-American Fertility," supported by a grant from the National Institute of Child Health and Human Development. John Meredith, a doctoral candidate in anthropology who also has a master's degree in Spanish, and I, an anthropologist and registered nurse, conducted these interviews. The words were transcribed from tapes by Wendy Redlinger, project secretary, and doctoral candidate in linguistics.

The manuscript was prepared using Dow Robinson's *Manual for Bilingual Dictionaries* (1969) as a guide. Paul and Shirley Turner's *Chontal to Spanish-English Dictionary* (1971) was our model. These two works suggested the need for sentences to illustrate word use. So the four of us combed our data to make sentences. All of us checked each entry, dividing final decisions as follows: Entries were chosen and sentences verified for accuracy of folk and official Western medical content by Kay, for syntax by Meredith, and for regionalisms by Raymond. Redlinger organized the entire manuscript. Camera-ready copy was typed by Joyce Drennen. The manuscript was prepared using funds from the Ethnosemantics grant.

We invite suggestions from our readers for new entries, corrections or deletions. We gratefully acknowledge the forebearance of Arthur Kay, Judi Meredith, Bruce Raymond, and Thomas Redlinger. Especial thanks to Gladys Sorensen, Dean of the College of Nursing, for it was her persistent encouragement that decided the creation of this book. We would also like to thank Vicente Acosta, Robert Bacalski, Dolores Brown, Frances Ríos, and Arnulfo Trejo for explanations and clarifications of medical terminology in southwestern American Spanish. A note of appreciation is also due the University of Arizona Press for effecting publication.

Margarita Kay

USE OF THE DICTIONARY

Spanish Section

Each entry is in bold-face type. In the Spanish-to-English section, verbs are given in the infinitive and labeled with the abbreviation *v*. Nouns are identified by gender, *m*. for masculine and *f*. for feminine. Adjectives are labeled *adj*. and adverbs, *adv*. When the entry is a phrase, there is no designation of part of speech.

If the entry is next labeled as *ethn*., the term is a folk designation. An equivalent in English is offered if possible. The Latin binomial is given for herbs.

The entry that is labeled *coll*. for colloquial is an extremely familiar term. It is given in the dictionary because it may be used by a patient. However, it is not suitable for the health worker to approach the patient with such a term.

The English translation follows, printed in italics. The word is then used in a sentence, as it might be stated by a patient, or by a health worker presenting information. The example sentence is then translated into English. If the word has a synonym, it is listed in parentheses, following the abbreviation *syn*.

English Section

In the English section, the word is identified by part of speech. The Spanish gloss follows, with gender of noun.

Abbreviations

adj.	adjective	m.	masculine
adv.	adverb	n.	noun
coll.	colloquial	pl.	plural
ethn.	ethnic	syn.	synonym
f.	feminine	v.	verb

Appendixes

Appendix A: Food Items

Appendix B: Kinship Terms

Appendix C: Other Useful Sources of Spanish Medical Terminology

Spanish to English

SPANISH
TO
ENGLISH

---

abdomen m. *abdomen*. Mucha gente usa el término 'estómago' para referirse al abdomen. *Many people use the term 'stomach' to refer to the abdomen.* (Syn: estómago)

abertura del paladar *cleft palate*. Cuando se opera de la abertura del paladar, la persona puede hablar normalmente. *After cleft palate surgery a person can speak normally.* (Syn: boquinete)

aborto (natural) *miscarriage*. Sufrió un aborto después de dos meses de embarazo. *She had a miscarriage after two months of pregnancy.* (Syn: mal parto)

aborto (provocado) *induced abortion*. Unas medicinas pueden provocar abortos. *Some medicines can induce abortions.*

abrir v. *to open*. Abra la boca, por favor. *Open your mouth, please.* —adj. abierto

absceso m. *abscess.* Mi hijo tiene un absceso en el cuello que no se le va. *My son has an abscess on the neck that will not go away.* (Syns: postema, apostema)

acabar v. *to experience orgasm, arrive at a climax.* Algunos creen que si acaban los dos juntos, la mujer va a salir embarazada. *Some believe that if both experience orgasm simultaneously, the wife will get pregnant.*

acabarse v. *to be used up, all gone.* Tengo que ir a la farmacia porque se acabaron las píldoras. *I have to go to the drugstore because the pills are all gone.*

acceso m. *attack.* Se me vino un acceso de tos. *I had a coughing attack.*

acedías f. *heartburn.* Uno tiene la tendencia a sufrir de acedías después de comer chile. *One has a tendency to suffer heartburn after eating chili.* (Syns: acidez, agruras del estómago)

aceite de comer *cooking oil (medicinally, olive oil).* Se le puso al niño algodoncitos con aceite de comer en los oídos dolorosos. *Cotton balls soaked in olive oil were put in the child's aching ears.*

acidez f. *heartburn.* See **acedías**.

acostarse v. *to lie down.* Si uno está cansado es buena idea acostarse. *If one is tired it is a good idea to lie down.*

acostumbrarse v. *to get used to.* Los diabéticos tienen que acostumbrarse a no comer el azúcar. *Diabetics have to get used to not eating sugar.*

acto sexual *sexual intercourse.* La vasectomía no afecta el acto sexual.
*Vasectomy does not affect the sexual
act.* (Syn: coito)

achaque m. *systemic weakness.* María ha
sufrido de achaques al corazón por dos
años. *Maria has had a problematic heart
for two years.*

adormecido, -a adj. (tener) *numb.* Tengo
adormecido el brazo. *My arm feels numb.*
—n. adormecimiento.

afectar v. *to affect.* Ciertas drogas afectan
la coordinación física. *Certain drugs
affect physical coordination.*

aflojar v. *to loosen.* Por favor, afloje el
cinto. *Please loosen your belt.*

aflojarse v. *to relax.* No es posible aflojarse
si uno está nervioso. *It's impossible to
relax if one is nervous.* (Syn: relajarse)

agarrar v. *to take hold of, to grab.* Agárrate
bien para que no te caigas del columpio.
*Hold on tight so that you will not fall
off the swing.*

agarrar v. (coll.) *to catch.* Agarró el
sarampión de su primo. *He caught the
measles from his cousin.* (Syn: pegarle a
uno)

agitado, -a adj. *agitated, upset.* Se puso
muy agitado cuando supo que tenía
cancer. *He got very upset when he
found out that he had cancer.*

agotado, -a adj. (sentirse *or* estar) *exhausted, fatigued.* Después de la operación, me sentí muy agotada. *I felt very exhausted after the operation.* —n. agotamiento.

agravarse v. *to get worse.* Con los años, se agravó su enfermedad. *With the years his sickness got worse.* (Syn: empeorarse)

agresivo, -a adj. *aggressive.* El alcohol le pone muy agresivo. *Alcohol makes him very aggressive.*

agruras del estómago f. pl. *heartburn.* A veces he sentido agruras en el estómago después de comer. *Sometimes I have had heartburn after eating.* (Syns: acedías, acidez)

agua f. (el) *water.* Es mejor beber agua purificada cuando uno viaja. *It is better to drink purified water when one travels.*

agua en el cerebro *water on the brain.* Los cirujanos pueden poner una sonda para sacar el agua del cerebro. *Surgeons can use a catheter to drain water on the brain.*

ahogarse v. *to drown; to choke.* Se ahogó porque no sabia nadar. *She drowned because she did not know how to swim.*

aire m. *air.* Para tener buen salud, se necesita aire puro. *In order to be healthy one needs pure air.*

aire m. (pasar) *gas.* Después de comer frijoles siempre paso aire. *After eating beans I always pass gas.* (Syns: gas, viento, pedo)

ajo m. (herb) *garlic (Allium sativum).* Used as a suppository in treatment of tripa ida.

alacrán m. *scorpion.* El alacrán es un insecto venenoso que vive en el desierto. *A scorpion is a poisonous insect of the desert.* (Syn: escorpión)

alambrito m. *I.U.D., coil, loop.* Se pone el alambrito en la matriz de la mujer. *The coil is put in the woman's uterus.* (Syns: coil, tubo de plástico, aparatito)

alcohol m. *alcohol.* Demasiado alcohol daña el hígado. *Too much alcohol harms the liver.*

alcoholismo m. *alcoholism.* El alcoholismo indica una debilidad del carácter. *Alcoholism shows weakness of character.*

aldilla f. *groin.* Una hernia en la aldilla causa mucho dolor. *A hernia in the groin is very painful.* (Syn: ingle)

alegre adj. *happy.* El parece alegre aunque esta padeciendo. *He seems happy even though he is suffering.* (Syn: feliz)

alferecía f. (ethn.) *convulsions resulting from febrile illness.* La alferecía puede ocurrir después del sarampión. *Convulsions resulting from fever can set in following measles.*

algodón m. *cotton.* Limpie la herida con algodón esterilizado. *Clean the wound with sterile cotton.*

alguate m. *cactus sticker.* Tenga cuidado con los alguates de los cactos. *Be careful with the cactus stickers.* (Syn: espina)

aliento m. (buen *or* mal) *breath.* El mal aliento puede indicar una infección. *Bad breath may indicate an infection.*

alimentación f. *nourishment.* Le dan caldo como alimentación. *He is given soup for nourishment.*

aliviar v. *to alleviate, soothe.* Hay cremas que pueden aliviar las quemaduras. *There are creams that can soothe burns.*

aliviarse v. *to get well.* Me alivié del catarro rápidamente. *I got over my cold quickly.* (Syn: sanarse)

almidón m. *starch.* El grano de trigo consiste por la mayor parte de almidón. *A grain of wheat consists primarily of starch.*

almorranas f. pl. *piles, hemorrhoids.* Después del embarazo, sufrí de almorranas. *After my pregnancy I suffered from hemorrhoids.*

alta presión *high blood pressure.* Demasiada sal en la comida puede causar alta presión. *Too much salt in food can bring on high blood pressure.*

alucinaciones f. pl. *hallucinations.* Ciertas drogas producen alucinaciones. *Certain drugs produce hallucinations.* (Syn: visiones)

amarillo, -a adj. *yellow.* La niña se puso amarilla a los tres días de edad. *The three-day-old baby girl turned yellow.*

amarrar los tubos *to tie the tubes, tubal ligation.* Después de amarrar los tubos no se puede volver a tener familia. *After tying the tubes one cannot have children again.*

amiba f. (var. of **ameba**) *amoeba.* La amiba puede causar disentería. *The amoeba can cause dysentery.*

amígdalas f. pl. *tonsils (rare).* Tiene pus en las amígdalas. *There is pus on the tonsils.* (Syn: anginas)

amnesia f. *amnesia.* La amnesia es la pérdida de la memoria. *Amnesia is memory loss.*

amodorrado, -a adj. *drowsy.* Ella se sintió muy amodorrada después del anestésico. *She felt very drowsy after the anaesthetic.*

ampolla f. *blister.* Los zapatos apretados me dieron ampollas. *The tight shoes gave me blisters.*

análisis m. *(laboratory) test.* El chequeo general incluye varios análisis. *A general checkup includes various analyses.*

análisis de *analysis of (blood, urine, etc.).* Se toma un análisis de la orina para ver si hay diabetes. *A urine sample is taken to see if there is diabetes.* (Syns: prueba, examen)

andar v. *to walk.* El bebé no puede andar todavía. *The baby cannot walk yet.* (Syn: caminar)

andar volado (coll.) *to go beserk; to be distracted.* Después del trauma emocional andaba volado. *After the emotional trauma he went beserk.*

anemia f. *anemia.* Cuando falta hierro en la sangre, hay anemia. *When the blood lacks iron, anemia occurs.* (Syns: sangre débil, sangre pobre)

animar v. *to encourage.* El esposo puede animar a la esposa cuando ella está dando a luz. *The husband may give encouragement to the wife when she is giving birth.*

anginas f. pl. *tonsils.* Ella tenía las anginas muy inflamadas. *Her tonsils were very inflamed.* (Syn: amígdalas)

angustia f. *anguish.* Sintió mucha angustia al saber que su esposo se había muerto. *She felt much anguish upon learning that her husband had died.*

anís m. (herb) *anise (Pimpinella anisum).* *Prepared as tea for treatment of colic.*

anormal adj. *abnormal.* Es anormal no querer comer. *It is abnormal not to want to eat.*

ansias f. pl. *anxiety.* El no estar seguro de sí mismo causa ansias. *Not being sure of oneself causes anxiety.* (Syn: ansiedad)

ansiedad f. *anxiety.* See **ansias.**

ansioso, -a adj. *anxious, worried.* Está muy ansioso pero sin razón. *He is very worried but without reason.*

anticonceptivo, -a adj. *contraceptive.* La pastilla anticonceptiva es un método de cuidarse muy popular. *The contraceptive pill is a popular method of birth control.*

anticonceptivo m. *contraceptive.* Los anticonceptivos ayudan a evitar el embarazo. *Contraceptives help avoid pregnancy.*

antiflogístico m. *antiphlogistic.* Vick's es un antiflogístico popular. *Vick's is a popular antiphlogistic.*

antojo m. *craving.* Muchas mujeres tienen antojos durante el embarazo. *Many women have cravings during their pregnancy.*

añil m. (herb) *bluing (Indigofera suffruticosa). Crushed and used as a treatment for* empacho.

aparatito m. *I.U.D., coil, loop.* El aparatito es un anticonceptivo que se pone en la matriz. *The I.U.D. is a contraceptive that is placed in the uterus.* (Syns: coil, tubo de plástico, alambrito)

apendicitis f. *appendicitis.* La gente cree que el comer las semillas de los chiles a veces causa la apendicitis. *People believe that eating chile seeds will sometimes cause appendicitis.*

apendis m. (var. of **apéndice**) *appendix.* El apendis es una parte de los intestinos. *The appendix is a part of the intestines.*

apestar v. *to stink.* El aliento puede apestar si uno no se lava los dientes regularmente. *The breath may stink if one does not brush his teeth regularly.* (Syn: heder)

apetito m. *appetite.* No tiene apetito porque siente náuseas. *He has a poor appetite because he feels nauseated.* (Syn: ganas de comer)

apostema f. *abscess.* La apostema es una infección de los tejidos debajo de la piel. *An abscess is an infection of tissues under the skin.* (Syns: absceso, postema)

apretar v. *to tighten.* Apriete los ojos, por favor. *Close your eyes tightly, please.*

aprovecharse v. (de) *to take advantage of.* La gente pobre debe aprovecharse de los cupones para alimentos. *Poor people should take advantage of food coupons.*

araña f. *spider.* Algunas arañas son venenosas. *Some spiders are poisonous.*

arañar v. (also **aruñar**) *to scratch.* El gato le arañó al niño. *The cat scratched the child.* (Syn: rasguñar, rascar)

arder v. *to burn.* Me ha estado ardiendo mucho la cortada. *The cut has been burning a great deal.*

ardor m. *burning sensation.* La señora siente un ardor en el estómago. *The lady feels a burning sensation in the stomach.*

ardor al orinar *burning on urination.* Un ardor al orinar indica una infección de la vejiga. *A burning sensation on urination indicates a bladder infection.*

arreglar v. *to mend, fix.* Es mejor arreglar su dentadura ahora que esperar y tener más complicaciones. *It is better to fix your teeth now than to wait and have more complications.* (Syn: componer)

arrugas f. pl. *wrinkles.* La vieja tiene arrugas en la cara. *The old lady has wrinkles in her face.*

arteria f. *artery.* Las arterias llevan la sangre del corazón al cuerpo. *The arteries carry the blood from the heart to the body.*

articulación f. *joint.* La artritis ocurre cuando hay inflamación de las articulaciones del cuerpo. *Arthritis occurs when there is inflammation of the joints of the body.* (Syn: coyuntura)

artritis f. *arthritis.* La inflamación de las coyuntutas cause la artritis. *Inflammation of the joints causes arthritis.*

aruñar v. *to scratch.* See **arañar.**

asco m. *revulsion, disgust.* La comida extraña le da asco. *The strange food revolts him.*

aseo m. *cleanliness.* El aseo personal es imperativo para la buena salud. *Personal hygiene is imperative to good health.*

aseo m. *perineal care.* El aseo es importante para que se sanen las puntadas. *Perineal care is important for the healing of stitches.*

asistir al parto *to deliver.* Una partera asistió al parto de mi hermana. *A midwife delivered my sister's baby.*

asqueroso, -a adj. *filthy.* La zanja asquerosa amenazaba la salud del barrio. *The filthy ditch threatened neighborhood health.* (Syn: inmundo)

astilla f. *sliver.* Le entraron astillas cuando jugaba béisbol con el bate viejo. *He got slivers when he played baseball with the old bat.*

asustarse v. *to become frightened.* El niño se asustó a causa del relámpago. *The child was frightened by the lightning.*

atarantarse v. *to become dizzy or light-headed.* Cuando uno se siente débil es muy fácil atarantarse. *When one feels weak it is very easy to become dizzy.*

ataque al corazón *heart attack, myocardial infarction.* Falleció de un ataque al corazón. *He died of a heart attack.* (Syn: infarto)

atorarse v. *to obstruct.* Un pedazo de hielo se le atoró la traquea. *A piece of ice obstructed his trachea.* (Syn: obstruir)

atole m. *corn starch gruel, a semisolid food prepared for infants and invalids, frequently flavored with fruit or berries.* Al niño le gusta el atole. *The child likes atole.*

atragantarse v. *to choke.* Los niños pueden atragantarse fácilmente si beben rápidamente. *Children can choke easily if they drink rapidly.* (Syn: ahogarse)

atrasado, -a adj. *late.* Una regla atrasada pueda indicar que una esté embarazada. *A late period may mean that one is pregnant.*

atrasado, -a n. *retarded (person).* Los atrasados se pueden educar por especialistas. *The mentally retarded can be educated by specialists.*

autorecetarse v. *to prescribe for oneself.* En casos graves es peligroso autorecetarse. *In serious cases it is dangerous to prescribe for oneself.*

avergonzarse v. *to be ashamed, embarrassed.* Muchas señoritas se avergüenzan durante los exámenes médicos. *Many young ladies are embarrassed during medical examinations.*

avispa f. *wasp.* La picada de la avispa puede ser muy seria. *The wasp sting may be very serious.*

axila f. *armpit.* Se puede medir la temperatura en la axila. *Temperature can be taken in the armpit.* (Syn: sobaco)

ayudar al parto (see **asistir al parto**) *to deliver.*

ayunar v. *to fast.* Los pacientes suelen ayunar antes de una operación. *Patients usually fast before an operation.*

azahar m. (herb) *orange blossom (Citrus aurantium). Prepared as a tea and used to treat heart and nerve disorders.*

azúcar en el orín *diabetes, sugar diabetes.* Es muy importante seguir un régimen médico para controlar el azúcar en el orin. *It's very important to follow a medical regime in order to control sugar diabetes.* (Syn: diabetes)

azul adj. *blue.* El niño se pone azul por falta de oxígeno. *The child turns blue from oxygen deficiency.*

B

babear v. *to drool.* Los niños babean mucho cuando les salen los dientes. *When children are teething, they drool a lot.*

bacín m. *bed pan.* Tráigame el bacín. *Bring me the bed pan.*

bajar de peso *to lose weight.* Durante la enfermedad él bajó mucho de peso. *During the illness, he lost a lot of weight.*

bajarle la regla *to flow (menstrual).* A las mujeres que usan la pastilla no les baja la regla tanto. *Women who use the pill do not flow as much.*

bala f. *bullet.* La bala le penetró el pecho. *The bullet penetrated the chest.*

balance m. (coll.) *balance.* Perdió su balance y se cayó. *She lost her balance and fell.* (Syn: equilibrio)

balazo m. *bullet wound.* Le dió un balazo en el pecho. *He shot him in the chest.*

bañarse v. *to bathe.* Necesita bañarse con agua tibia para bajar la calentura. *He needs to bathe with warm water to lower his temperature.*

baño m. *bath.* La madre da un baño al bebé. *The mother gives a bath to the baby.*

baño m. *bathroom.* La mujer embarazada tiene que ir al baño muy de seguido. *The pregnant woman has to go to the bathroom frequently.*

baño de toalla m. *sponge bath.* Después de la operación solamente podía tomar baños de toalla. *After the operation he could only take sponge baths.*

barba f. *chin; beard.* Cuando se paró el carro de golpe él se lastimó la barba. *When the car suddenly stopped he hurt his chin.* (Syn: piocha)

barba de elote (herb) *corn tassel (Zea mays).* Prepared as a tea and used to treat kidney ailments.

barriga f. (coll.) *belly, tummy.* Cuando tenía diarrea me dolía la barriga. *When I had diarrhea my belly hurt.* (Syn: panza)

basca f. *vomitus,* n. La basca salió amarilla. *The vomitus came out yellow.* (Syn: vómito)

bazo m. *spleen.* Después del choque tuvieron que sacarle el bazo al motociclista. *After his crash they had to remove the motorcyclist's spleen.*

bebé m. *baby.* Es mejor criar al bebé con pecho. *It is best to breast feed the baby.* (Syn: criatura, "baby")

beber v. *to drink.* Cuando uno tiene la gripe es importante beber muchos líquidos. *When one has the flu it is important to drink a lot of liquid.* (Syn: tomar)

biberón m. *nursing bottle.* Para suplementar la leche de la madre, se puede usar el biberón. *To supplement mother's milk one can use a nursing bottle.* (Syns: mamadera, tetera, botella)

bilis f. (lay) *gall bladder disease, cholecystitis.* Cuando uno sufre de la bilis a veces hay que sacar la vesícula biliar. *When one suffers from cholecystitis sometimes it is necessary to remove the gall bladder.* (Syn: dolor de la vesícula biliar, mal de hiel)

bilis f. (ethn.) *bile (secretion of gall bladder, believed to be stimulated by anger).* El mucho coraje causa que se reviente la hiel y que se derrame la bilis. *Anger causes the gall bladder to burst and bile to spill.*

bilma f. (ethn.) *cast made of leaves, etc.* En los ranchos solían hacer bilmas de hojas de álamo. *On ranches they used to make casts from cottonwood leaves.*

biopsia f. *biopsy.* Tomaron una biopsia para ver si el tumor era maligno. *They did a biopsy in order to see if the tumor was malignant.*

bizco, -a adj. *cross-eyed.* El niño bizco nació así. *The cross-eyed child was born that way.*

blanco, -a adj. *white.* Un desecho blanco y espeso puede significar una infección de la vagina. *A thick white discharge may indicate a vaginal infection.*

bobito m. *eye gnat (hippelates).* Los bobitos molestan los ojos. *Gnats bother the eyes.*

boca f. *mouth.* Abra la boca, por favor. *Please open your mouth.*

boca abajo *face down.* Acuéstese boca abajo, por favor. *Please lie face down.*

boca arriba *face up.* Por favor acuéstese boca arriba. *Please lie down face up.*

boca del estómago *esophagus, gullet.* El ácido quema la boca del estómago. *Acid burns the esophagus.* (Syns: esófago, tragante)

bocio m. *goiter.* El bocio es el engrandeci-
miento de la tiroides. *Goiter is the
enlargement of the thyroid.* (Syn:
buche)

bolas f. pl. *balls, knots, tissue swelling. May
be applied to tonsils, lymph glands, and
mumps.* Dicen que bolas en la nuca
vienen de nerviosidad. *They say knots
come in the back of the neck from
nervousness.*

boldo m. (herb) *bold (Puemus boldus).
Prepared as a tea and used to aid digestion.*

bolita f. *lump.* El doctor le examinó los
pechos para ver si tenía bolitas. *The
doctor felt her breasts for lumps.* (Syn:
endurecimiento)

bolsa de aguas *bag of waters, amniotic sac.*
El feto crece en la bolsa de aguas. *The
fetus grows in the bag of waters.*

boquinete m. *cleft palate.* Cuando uno nace
con boquinete no es posible hablar clara-
mente. *When one is born with a cleft
palate he can't speak clearly.* (Syn:
abertura del paladar)

borracho, -a adj. *drunk.* El perdió su
trabajo porque llegó borracho a la
oficina. *He lost his job because he
arrived drunk at the office.*

borraja f. (herb) *borage (Borago officinalis).
Prepared as a tea and used to treat
cough.*

bostezar v. *to yawn.* Cuando uno tiene sueño bosteza muy de seguido. *When one is sleepy he yawns frequently.*

botella f. *bottle; nursing bottle.* En vez de darle el pecho al bebé, la madre le da la botella. *Instead of breast feeding the baby, the mother gives him the bottle.*

botica f. *drugstore.* Venden medicinas en las boticas. *They sell medicines in drugstores.* (Syn: farmacia)

brazo m. *arm.* Muchas inyecciones se dan en el brazo. *Many shots are given in the arm.*

bronquitis f. *bronchitis.* Tiene tos porque padece de bronquitis. *He has a cough because he is suffering from bronchitis.*

brotar v. *to break out.* Le brotó un sarpullido a la criatura. *The baby broke out in a rash.*

brujo, -a n. *witch.* Una bruja usa magia negra para causar maldades. *A witch uses black magic to cause evil.*

buche m. (coll.) *goiter.* Al bocio se le llama buche en Sonora. *Goiter is called* buche *in Sonora.* (Syn: bocio)

bueno, -a adj. *good.* La medicina es muy buena. *The medicine is very good.*

buqui, -a n. (ethn.) *child.* 'Buqui' es un modismo sonorense para muchacho. Buqui *is a Sonoran idiom for boy.*

C

cabecita de vena *angioma.* Las cabecitas de vena aparecen como puntos rojos en la piel. *Angiomata appear like red spots on the skin.*

cabello m. *hair (of head).* Es necesario lavarse el cabello muy bien para evitar la caspa. *It is necessary to wash one's hair very well to avoid dandruff.* (Syn: pelo)

cabeza f. *head.* ¿Le duele la cabeza? *Does your head hurt?*

caca f. (hacer) *feces (translingual term of children).* El niño ya hace caca en el excusado. *The baby already makes caca in the toilet.*

caca aguada *mushy stool.* Si el niño tiene la caca aguada, él está enfermo. *If the child has a mushy stool he is sick.* (Syn: escremento aguado)

cachetar v. *to slap the face.* Voy a cachetar a ese niño travieso. *I'm going to slap that mischievous child.*

cachete m. (coll.) *cheek.* Tiene un rasguño en el cachete. *He has a scratch on his cheek.* (Syn: mejilla)

cada ocho días *once a week, each week, weekly.* Ud. debe pesarse cada ocho días para ver si ha perdido peso. *You should weigh yourself weekly to see if you have lost weight.* (Syns: cada semana, semanalmente)

cada semana *weekly.* See **cada ocho dias.**

cadera f. *hip, pelvis.* El parto fue difícil porque tiene la cadera estrecha. *The delivery was difficult because she has a narrow pelvis.*

cadera dislocada de nacimiento *congenital hip, congenital dislocation of the hip.* La cadera dislocada de nacimiento salió en el rayo equis. *The congenital dislocation of the hip showed up in the X ray.*

caer bien *to agree with.* Esa comida no me cayó bien y ahora me duele el estómago. *That food didn't agree with me and now my stomach hurts.*

caer mal *to disagree with one.* Sé que me cae mal la pastilla porque me hace vomitar. *I know the pill disagrees with me because it makes me vomit.*

caerse v. *to fall down.* Los ancianos deben cuidarse para no caerse y lastimarse. *Old people should be careful not to fall down and hurt themselves.*

calambre m. *muscle cramp*. Los calambres de las piernas son comunes cuando se nada. *Leg cramps are common when one is swimming.*

cálculo m. *stone, calculus*. Los cálculos de la vesícula biliar causan mucho dolor. *Gall bladder stones cause much pain.* (Syn: piedra)

calentura f. *fever, temperature*. A veces las criaturas tienen calentura cuando les salen los dientes. *Sometimes babies have a fever when they are teething.* (Syn: fiebre)

caliente adj. *hot*. Su piel estaba muy caliente a causa de la fiebre. *Her skin was very hot on account of the fever.*

calilla f. *suppository*. La madre puso una calilla en el niño porque él no obraba. *The mother put a suppository in the child because he hadn't moved his bowels.* (Syn: supositorio)

calmante m. *tranquilizer*. Algunas personas toman calmantes para tranquilizar los nervios. *Some people take tranquilizers to calm their nerves.* (Syn: tranquilizador)

calofrío m. *hot flash*. Cuando llegó al cambio de vida experimentó calofríos. *When she reached the change of life, she experienced hot flashes.*

calor m. *heat*. Se desmayó por el calor. *She fainted because of the heat.*

calores m. pl. *hot flashes*. See **calofrío**.

calvo, -a adj. *bald*. La cabeza calva debe de protegerse del sol. *Bald heads should be protected from the sun.*

callarse *to quiet down*. La criatura se calló después de que le dieron la mamadera. *The baby quieted down after they gave it the bottle.*

callo m. *callus, corn*. Los diabéticos no deben de operar sus propios callos. *Diabetics should not operate on their own calluses.*

cambiar v. *to change*. A las criaturas se les cambia la zapeta muchas veces diariamente. *One changes babies' diapers several times daily.*

cambio de vida *change of life, menopause*. La mujer puede empezar el cambio de vida a los cuarenta años de edad. *A woman can begin the change of life at forty*. (Syn: menopausia)

caminar v. *to walk*. Es bueno caminar diariamente. *It's good to walk daily*. (Syn: andar)

campanilla f. *uvula*. La campanilla del paladar a veces se hincha. *The uvula of the palate sometimes swells*. (Syn: úvula)

canela f. (herb) *cinnamon (Cinnamomum zeylanicum). Prepared as a tea and used to treat cough.*

cansancio m. *tiredness, fatigue.* Después de un día largo de trabajo es común el cansancio. *After a long day of work tiredness is common.* (Syn: fatiga)

cansarse v. *to tire, to get tired.* El enfermo se cansa fácilmente. *The sick person tires easily.*

canutillo m. (herb) *mormon tea (Ephedra trifurca). Prepared as a tea and used to treat anemia.*

capirotada f. *Mexican bread pudding.* Se alternan capas de pan, queso, nueces y pasas, se agrega vino y se pone al horno para hacer capirotada. *Alternate layers of bread, cheese and raisins, add wine and bake to make* capirotada.

cápsula f. *capsule.* Muchas medicinas vienen en cápsulas. *Many medicines come in capsules.*

cara f. *face.* Las caras de los adolescentes suelen tener granos. *Adolescents' faces often have pimples.*

carencia f. *deficiency, lack.* La carencia de niacina causa la pelagra. *Lack of niacin causes pellagra.* (Syn: deficiencia)

carnal m. & f. *blood relative (by extension, close friend).* El es mi carnal. *He is my blood relative.*

carne f. *flesh.* El fuego le quemó la carne del brazo. *The fire burned the flesh on his arm.*

carnosidad del ojo *fleshy growth of eye, pterigium.* Es común la carnosidad del ojo en las tortilleras. *Pterigia are common in people who make tortillas.*

casarse v. (con) *to marry.* Se casó con ella aunque era su sobrina. *He married her even though she was his niece.*

casco de la cabeza *scalp.* Hay que mantener el casco de la cabeza limpio para evitar la caspa. *It is necessary to keep one's scalp clean to avoid dandruff.*

caspa f. *dandruff.* La caspa puede ser el resultado de no lavarse bien el cabello. *Dandruff can be the result of not washing one's hair well.*

cataplasmo m. *medicated compress.* Antes, usaban hediondilla como cataplasmo en la pierna. *Formerly they used creosote as a medicated compress on the leg.*

catarata f. *cataract.* Hay cataratas que necesitan operarse para evitar la ceguera. *There are cataracts that need to be operated on to prevent blindness.* (Syn: nube del ojo)

catarro m. *common cold.* El catarro se puede confundir con una alergia crónica. *A cold can be confused with a chronic allergy.* (Syn: resfriado)

causar v. *to cause.* El comer demasiado causa gordura. *Eating too much causes obesity.*

ceguera f. *blindness.* Las nubes en los ojos pueden causar ceguera. *Cataracts can cause blindness.*

ceja f. *eyebrow.* Tiene las cejas gruesas. *He has thick eyebrows.*

celoso, -a adj. *jealous.* Cuando llegó el segundo hijo, se puso celoso el primero. *When the second child arrived, the first became jealous.* (Syn: tener celos)

centro de salud *health department.* Dan varias clases de inmunización en los centros de salud. *They give various kinds of immunization at health departments.*

cepillo m. *brush.* Limpia sus dientes con un cepillo. *He cleans his teeth with a brush.* —v. cepillar.

cera f. *wax (cerumen).* Es mala idea sacarse la cera de los oídos. *It is a bad idea to take the wax out of your ears.*

cerebro m. *brain, cerebrium.* Muchas veces es posible quitar tumores del cerebro. *It is often possible to remove brain tumors.*

cerebro m. (lay) *occiput, back of neck.* Tengo el cerebro tieso. *I have a stiff neck.*

cerrar v. *close.* Cierre los ojos. *Close your eyes.*

cicatriz f. *scar.* La herida dejó una cicatriz muy obvia. *The wound left a very obvious scar.*

ciempiés m. *centipede.* El ciempiés del desierto es un insecto no muy venenoso. *The desert centipede is a mildly poisonous insect.*

cilantro m. (herb) *coriander (Coriandum sativum).* Prepared as a tea and used to bring on a delayed menstrual period.

cintura f. *waist.* Por favor quítese la ropa de la cintura para abajo (arriba). *Please take off your clothes from the waist down (up).*

cintura f. (lay) *small of back.* El dolor de la cintura ocurre a causa del mal de riñón. *Pain in the back is caused by kidney disease.*

cirujano, -a n. *surgeon.* Un cirujano es un médico que sabe operar. *A surgeon is a doctor who knows how to operate.*

cita f. *appointment.* Tengo una cita con el médico a la una. *I have an appointment with the doctor at one o'clock.*

clara f. *white (of egg).* La clara del huevo contiene proteína. *The white of the egg contains protein.*

claro, -a adj. *clear, glairy.* La flema clara puede ser una indicación de jey fiver. *Clear mucus may be an indication of hay fever.*

clavícula f. *collar bone, clavicle.* Cuando está naciendo el niño, puede quebrarse su clavícula. *When the infant is being delivered his clavicle may be broken.*

cleptómano, -a n. *kleptomaniac.* El cleptómano no sabe por qué roba. *The kleptomaniac does not know why he steals.*

clitoris m. *clitoris.* La mujer tradicional no se da cuenta que tiene clitoris hasta que empieza la actividad sexual. *The old-fashioned woman does not realize she has a clitoris until she begins sexual activity.* (Syn: pepa)

coágulo m. *blood clot, thrombus.* Es peligroso tomar la pastilla cuando uno tiene la propensidad a tener coágulos. *It is dangerous to take the pill when one has a propensity to have blood clots.* (Syns: cuajarón, cuajo)

cobrar v. *to charge.* El médico cobra diez dólares por la visita. *The doctor charges ten dollars a visit.*

cócciz m. *tailbone, coccyx.* El cócciz es el último hueso de la columna vertebral. *The coccyx is the last bone of the vertebral column.* (Syn: rabadilla)

cocido, -a adj. *cooked.* Las verduras cocidas tiene menos vitamina C que las verduras crudas. *Cooked vegetables contain less vitamin C than raw vegetables.*

coco m. *hurt, injury (term generally used by young children).* Mamá, tengo un coco en la rodilla. *Mama, I have a hurt on my knee.* (Syns: herida, lastimadura)

cocolmeca f. (herb) *sarsaparilla (Smilax mexicana). Prepared as a tea and used to treat kidney ailments.*

cochinada f. *junk.* Los niños comen muchas cochinadas. *Children eat a iot of junk.*

codo m. *elbow.* Suelen poner sueros en la vena del dobladillo del codo. *They put solutions in the vein in the crook of the elbow.*

coil m. *I.U.D., coil, loop.* Muchas mujeres prefieren el coil como método anticonceptivo. *Many women prefer the coil as a contraceptive method.* (Syns: tubo de plástico, alambrito, aparatito)

coito m. *coitus, sexual intercourse.* Coito es la palabra técnica para estar con el esposo. *Coitus is the technical word for sexual intercourse.* (Syn: acto sexual)

cojear v. *to limp.* El niño cojeaba porque tenía quebrada una pierna. *The child was limping because he had a broken leg.*

cojo, -a adj. *lame, crippled.* La guerra dejó al hombre cojo. *The war left the man crippled.*

colapso nervioso *nervous breakdown.* La mucha preocupación puede resultar en un colapso nervioso. *Excessive worry can cause a nervous breakdown.*

cólico m. *colic, severe abdominal cramps.* Se da manzanilla a las criaturas cuando sufren de cólico. *Camomile tea is given to babies with colic.*

colocar v. *to place.* Se coloca el aparatito en la matriz. *The I.U.D. is placed in the uterus.*

colorado, -a adj. *red.* Los ojos están colorados porque están infectados. *His eyes are red because they are infected.*

comadrona f. *midwife (empiric), "granny."* La comadrona aprendió su profesión de su madre. *The midwife learned her work from her mother.*

comezón f. *itching, pruritis.* Las picadas de mosquito causan comezones. *Mosquito bites cause itching.* (Syn: rasquera)

comodidad f. *convenience, comfort.* Los ricos tienen muchas comodidades en sus casas. *Rich people have many conveniences in their homes.*

comodidades f. pl. *restrooms.* Han instalado comodidades en muchos parques. *Restrooms have been installed in many parks.*

complejo m. *complex.* Su baja estatura le
ha dado un complejo de inferioridad.
*His short stature has given him an inferi-
ority complex.*

complicación f. *complication.* La pulmonía
puede ser una complicación del catarro.
*Pneumonia can be a complication of a
cold.*

componer v. (ethn.) *to mend, fix (folk
prenatal treatment).* Voy con la sobadora para que me componga. *I am going
to the masseuse so that she can fix the
position of the fetus.*

componerse v. *to mend; to get well.* Tiene
que quedarse en la cama para que su
pierna quebrada se componga. *You have
to stay in bed so that your broken leg
will mend.*

compresa f. *compress.* Se usan compresas
frías en las puntas infectadas. *Cold com-
presses are used on infected stitches.*

condición del tiempo *seasonal sickness.* Jey
fiver es una condición del tiempo
porque no pega a uno todo el año. *Hay
fever is a seasonal illness because it does
not attack all year.*

condón m. *condom, prophylactic, rubber.*
Muchos hombres usan los condones
como anticonceptivos. *Many men use
condoms as contraceptives.* (Syns: hule,
preservativo)

congestion de (lay) *congestion of, dysfunction of . . . believed due to increase of blood, mucus, etc. Term applied to head, chest, stomach, etc.* La medicina dada por vapor alivia la congestión del pecho. *Medicine administered by inhalation relieves chest congestion.*

congoja f. *tightness, pressure, anguish.* Sintió congoja en el pecho al subir las escaleras. *He felt pressure in his chest when climbing stairs.*

consolar v. *to console.* El sacerdote consoló al padre cuando murió su hijo. *The Priest consoled the father when his son died.*

constipado -a adj. *congested.* El niño amaneció muy constipado a causa del catarro. *The child awakened very congested from a cold.*

contagioso, -a adj. *contagious.* El sarampión es contagioso. *Measles are contagious.* (Syn: pegajoso)

contento, -a adj. *content, satisfied.* Fue contento con la atención que le dieron en el hospital. *He was satisfied with the attention they gave him in the hospital.*

contra prep. *against.* Empuje contra mi mano. *Push against my hand.*

convulsiones f. pl. *convulsions, fits.* La epilepsia causa convulsiones. *Epilepsy causes convulsions.*

coraje m. (dar, sentir) *anger.* Le dió mucho coraje que le cobraran tanto por el hospital. *He became furious when he found out he had been charged so much by the hospital.* (Syn: rabia)

coraje m. (ethn.) *anger (pathological condition believed to cause miscarriage, spoil breast milk, etc.).* La mujer creía que habia perdido al niño por coraje. *The woman believed that she had lost the baby from (pathological) anger.*

corazón m. *heart.* El corazón hace circular la sangre. *The heart makes the blood circulate.*

corazón grande *enlarged heart.* El corazón grande es el resultado de demasiada actividad del mismo. *An enlarged heart is the result of its overactivity.*

corona f. *crown (of the head).* Por lo general, la corona de la cabeza de un bebé es blanda. *Generally, the crown of a baby's head is soft.*

coronilla f. *crown (of the head).* See **corona.**

correr v. *to run.* El correr diariamente es bueno para la salud. *It is good for the health to run daily.*

cortada f. *cut, laceration, incision.* La cortada en la pierna se había infectado. *The cut on the leg had become infected.*

cortar v. *to cut.* El muchacho se cortó la mano. *The boy cut his hand.*

corto de respiración *short of breath, dyspneic.* Después del infarto, Papá estuvo corto de respiración. *After the infarct, Daddy was short of breath.* (Syn: dificultad al respirar)

costado m. *side of the body.* La señora tenía un dolor en el costado. *The lady had a pain in her side.*

cosquillas f. pl. (hacer) *to tickle.* El demasiado hacer cosquillas a los niños puede ser dañoso. *Tickling children too much can be dangerous.*

costilla f. *rib.* Al caerse, el niño se rompió una costilla. *On falling, the child broke a rib.*

costillas f. pl. *rib cage.* Una de las funciones de las costillas es proteger los pulmones. *One of the functions of the rib cage is to protect the lungs.*

costra f. *scab.* Es mejor dejar que una costra se caiga por sí sola. *It is better to let a scab fall off by itself.*

costumbre, f. *custom, habit.* El hombre tiene que cambiar sus costumbres perezosas. *The man must change his lazy habits.*

coyuntura f. *joint.* A los viejos les suelen doler las coyunturas a causa de los depósitos que se forman allí. *Old people usually have joint pains caused by precipitations.* (Syn: articulación)

cráneo m. *skull, cranium.* El cráneo protege el cerebro. *The skull protects the brain.*

crecer v. *to grow.* La alimentación es muy importante para garantizar que la criatura crezca bien. *Nourishment is important for the child to grow well.*

criar v. *to raise, rear.* Es importante criar a un niño bien para que sepa portarse bien. *It is important to raise a child well so that he will know how to behave properly.*

criar con pecho *breast feed.* La tendencia de hoy es de no criar a los bebés con pecho. *The tendency today is not to breast feed.* (Syns: dar de pecho, dar de mamar)

criatura f. *baby; fetus.* La mujer sintió los movimientos de la criatura en su vientre. *The woman felt the movements of the baby in her belly.* (Syns: bebé, "baby")

crisis nerviosa f. *anxiety attack.* Se preocupaba tanto con los problemas que tuvo una crisis nerviosa. *She worried about her problems so much that she had an anxiety attack.*

crónico, -a adj. *chronic.* La artritis es una enfermedad cronica. *Arthritis is a chronic disease.*

cruda f. *hangover.* La cruda es el resultado de haber tomado mucho licor la noche anterior. *A hangover is a result of having drunk a lot of alcohol the previous night.*

crudo, -a adj. *raw.* Las verduras crudas son buenas para la salud. *Raw vegetables are good for your health.*

cuadril m. *hip, pelvis (of animal familiarly applied to people).* El vaquero se quebró el cuadril al caerse del caballo. *The cowboy broke his hip by falling from the horse.*

cuajarón m. *blood clot, thrombus.* El enfermo escupió un cuajarón de sangre. *The sick man spat up a blood clot.* (Syns: coágulo, cuajo)

cuajo m. *blood clot, thrombus.* See **cuajarón**.

cuarentena f. (ethn.) *forty days following parturition, puerperium.* Antes, las mujeres tenían que evitar baños y algunos alimentos durante la cuarentena. *Previously, women had to avoid baths and some foods during the cuarentena.* (Syn: dieta)

cuate, -a n. *twin.* Los cuates idénticos se parecen el uno al otro. *Identical twins look alike.* (Syn: gemelo)

cucaracha f. *cockroach.* La cucaracha lleva microbios en sus patas. *The cockroach carries germs on its legs.*

cucharada f. *tablespoonful; liquid (medical) preparations.* Muchas medicinas líquidas se toman por cucharadas. *Many liquid medicines are taken by tablespoonfuls.*

cucharadita f. *teaspoonful.* Puso una cucharadita de azúcar en el café. *He put a teaspoonful of sugar in his coffee.*

cuello m. *front part of neck.* Las bolas en el cuello pueden señalar una infección de la garganta. *Lumps in the neck may indicate a throat infection.*

cuello de la matriz *cervix.* El diafragma tapa el cuello de la matriz. *The diaphragm covers the cervix.*

cuero m. (coll.) *skin.* La gente que está al sol mucho, tiene el cuero muy grueso. *People who are in the sun a great deal have a thick skin.*

cuidado prenatal *prenatal care.* Es importante ir al médico para el cuidado prenatal. *It is important to go to the doctor for prenatal care.*

cuidarse v. *to take care of (oneself), to take care not to get pregnant.* Mi esposa se cuida con la pastilla. *My wife uses the pill to avoid pregnancy.*

culebra f. *snake.* Las culebras venenosas son peligrosas. *Poisonous snakes are dangerous.* (Syn: víbora)

cuna f. *crib.* Los bebés duermen en una cuna. *Babies sleep in a crib.*

cundir v. *to spread.* La infección cundió porque no se limpió la herida. *The infection spread because the wound was not cleaned.*

curandero -a n. *healer.* El curandero conoce yerbas medicinales; sabe rezos y daños también. *The curandero knows medicinal herbs; prayers and hexes as well.*

cutis m. *complexion, skin of face.* Es importante proteger el cutis del sol. *It is important to protect the skin from the sun.*

Ch

chamaco, -a n. *kid, boy (girl).* El chamaco se sintió orgulloso cuando le empezó a crecer la barba. *The kid felt proud when his beard began to grow.*

chanza f. *mumps.* Es peligroso que le pegue la chanza a un hombre maduro. *It is dangerous for a grown man to get mumps.* (Syn: paperas)

charlatán m. *quack, charlatan.* Los charlatanes suelen saber muy poco acerca de la medicina. *Quacks usually know very little about medicine.* (Syn: merolico)

chequeo general médico *general checkup.* Es buena idea tener chequeo general médico para no enfermarse. *It is a good idea to have a general checkup so as to not get sick.*

chicura f. (herb) *ragweed (Ambrosia ambrocoides). Roots are made into solution for use in douching.*

chichis f. (coll.) *breasts.* Antes de la regla las chichis se engrandecen. *Before the menstrual period the breasts enlarge.* (Syns: pecho, teta)

chichón m. *bump or lump on the head.* Le salió un chichón después de que se golpeó la cabeza. *He got a lump after he hit his head.*

chiflar v. *to whistle; to wheeze.* Se puede oír el chiflar del asmático. *One can hear the wheezing of the asthmatic.* (Syn: silbar)

chilete m. (herb) *chilipiquin (Capsicum baccatum). Fried in oil and used as drops in treatment of earaches.*

chinche f. *bedbug.* En tiempos pasados las chinches eran muy comunes. *In previous times bedbugs were very common.*

chípili adj. *a spoiled or overindulged child.* Una criatura chípili puede llegar a ser un adulto con muchos problemas. *A spoiled child can turn out to be an adult with problems.* (Syns: mimado, echado a perder)

chorro m. *gush or spurt of fluid.* Cuando se cortó la arteria salió un chorro de sangre. *When he cut the artery, blood spurted out.*

chorro m. (coll.) *euphemism for gonorrhea.* El soldado le dió el chorro a la prostituta. *The soldier gave gonorrhea to the prostitute.* (Syns: gonorrea, purgación)

chot m. *shot, injection.* El doctor le dió un chot para curarle la gonorrea. *The doctor gave him a shot to cure him of gonorrhea.* (Syn: inyección)

choque m. *collision, impact.* Hubo una muerte a causa del choque automovilístico. *There was a death because of the automobile collision.*

choque m. *shock, trauma.* Sufrió un choque emocional cuando murió su madre. *He suffered an emotional shock when his mother died.* (Syn: susto)

chupar v. *to suck.* Los bebés nacen sabiendo chupar la leche. *Babies are born knowing how to suck milk.*

D

damiana f. (herb) *damiana (Turnera diffusa). Prepared as a solution and either drunk or used in a douche for treatment of* frío en la matriz.

daños m. pl. (ethn.) *includes a wide variety of physical symptoms that are unresponsive to medical treatment and are therefore attributed to witchcraft, hexes.* La mujer usó hechicería para hacer daños a su novio infiel. *The woman used witchcraft to harm her unfaithful lover.*

dañar v. *to harm.* El alcohol puede dañar el hígado. *Alcohol may be injurious to the liver.*

dañoso, -a adj. *injurious, harmful.* Demasiada comida puede ser dañosa. *Too much food can be injurious.*

dar de mamar v. *breast feed.* See **dar de pecho.**

dar a luz *to give birth.* El embarazo termina cuando se da a luz a la criatura. *Pregnancy ends when one gives birth to a child.* (Syn: sanar)

dar de pecho *breast feed.* Es más saludable para la criatura si uno le da de pecho. *It is healthier for the baby if one breast feeds it.* (Syns: criar con pecho, dar de mamar)

darse cuenta de *to realize.* Me dí cuenta de que el niño tenía fiebre cuando le tenté la frente. *I realized the child had a fever when I felt his forehead.*

darse en (el) v. *to bump.* El niño se dió en la cabeza con la mesa. *The child bumped his head on the table.*

débil adj. *weak.* La señora quedó débil después de la operación. *The woman remained weak after the operation.*

dedo m. *finger; toe.* Los dedos de los pies son más cortos que los dedos de las manos. *Toes are shorter than fingers.*

dedo gordo *thumb; great toe.* El niño se chupó el dedo gordo hasta los dos años de edad. *The child sucked his thumb until he was two years old.*

defecto de nacimiento *congenital malformation.* Ciertas drogas pueden causar defectos de nacimiento. *Certain drugs can cause congenital malformations.* (Syns: deformidad, deformación congénita)

deficiencia f. *deficiency, lack.* En los países subdesarrollados hay muchas personas con deficiencias nutritivas. *In undeveloped countries there are many persons with nutritional deficiencies.* (Syn: carencia)

deformación congénita congenital malformation. See **defecto de nacimiento.** (Syn: deformidad)

deformidad f. *congenital malformation.* See **defecto de nacimiento.** (Syn: deformación congénita)

delgadez f. *thinness.* La delgadez puede ocurrir a causa de la tuberculosis. *Thinness can be caused by tuberculosis.*

delirio m. *delirium.* La fiebre le causó delirio. *His fever caused delirium.* (Syn: desvarío)

demasiado adv. *too much; too . . .* ¡Señor, Ud. come demasiado . . . ! *Mister, you eat too much!*

dentadura f. *denture, set of teeth.* La dentadura artificial cuesta mucho. *False dentures cost a lot.*

dentición f. (lay) *teething, eruption of the teeth (physiological process is seen as period of illness).* Durante la dentición el niño tuvo diarrea. *While teething, the child had diarrhea.* (Syn: salida de los dientes)

dentro de prep. *inside.* El doctor puso el coil dentro de la matriz. *The doctor put the coil inside the uterus.*

deposición f. *bowel movement, stool, feces.* El enfermito hace muchas deposiciones. *The sick child has many bowel movements.*

derecho, -a adj. *right.* Muéstreme la mano derecha, por favor. *Show me your right hand, please.*

derecho adv. *straight ahead.* Mire derecho, por favor. *Look straight ahead, please.*

derramar v. *to pour, spill; to shed (blood).* Después del aborto la señora derramó mucha sangre. *After the miscarriage the woman shed a lot of blood.*

derrame del cerebro *stroke, C.V.A., cerebral hemorrhage.* Después que tuvo un derrame del cerebro quedó paralizada de la mano izquierda. *After she had a stroke her left hand remained paralyzed.* (Syns: embolio, estroc)

desarrollarse v. *to develop.* Los niños se desarrollan con rapidez si tienen comida adecuada. *Children develop rapidly if they have adequate food.*

descalzo, -a adj. *barefoot.* Alguna gente cree que si uno anda descalzo, le van a inflamar las anginas. *Some people believe that if one goes barefoot, his tonsils will become inflamed.*

descansar v. *to rest.* Los pacientes necesitan descansar mucho después de una operación. *Patients need to rest a lot after an operation.*

descanso m. *rest.* El señor necesitó mucho descanso después de su operación. *The man needed a lot of rest after his operation.*

descompostura f. *displacement.* La sobadora arregló la descompostura del hueso.
The sobadora *fixed the displacement of
the bone.*

desecho m. *discharge; menstrual discharge:
lochia.* El desecho después del parto
dura unas seis semanas. *The postpartum
discharge lasts up to about six weeks.*
(Syn: flujo)

deshidratar v. *dehydrate.* Con mucha
diarrea la criatura se deshidrata rápidamente. *With diarrhea, a child dehydrates
rapidly.*

desmayarse v. *to faint.* Antes las señoritas
solían desmayarse muy frecuentemente.
Young ladies used to faint very often.

desnutrido, -a adj. *undernourished.* A la
criatura desnutrida no puede combatir
infecciones. *The undernourished child
cannot fight infections.*

desombligado, -a adj. See **estar desombligado**.

destete m. *weaning.* Cuando se rechaza el
biberón es tiempo para el destete. *When
the bottle is refused it is time for weaning.* —v. destetar.

desvarío m. *delirium.* No sabe donde está porque padece de desvarío. *He does not know where he is because he is suffering from delirium.* (Syn: delirio)

desvestirse v. *to undress.* Señora, por favor desvístase de la cintura para arriba. *Ma'am, please undress from the waist up.* (Syn: quitarse la ropa)

diabetes f. (also diabetis) *diabetes, sugar diabetes.* Un síntoma de la diabetes es el exceso de azúcar en la sangre. *A symptom of diabetes is excess sugar in the blood.*

diafragma m. *diaphragm; vaginal diaphragm.* El diafragma es un método anticonceptivo. *The diaphragm is a contraceptive device.*

diarrea f. *diarrhea.* Le dió diarrea porque había comido carne podrida. *He had diarrhea because he had eaten rotten meat.* (Syns: excremento suelto, soltura)

dicipela f. (var. of ericipela: old) *erysipelas.* La dicipela es una enfermedad contagiosa de la piel. *Erysipelas is a contagious skin disease.*

diente m. *tooth.* Los dientes del niño no han brotado todavía. *The child's teeth have not erupted yet.*

dieta f. *diet.* La leche es importante en la dieta del niño. *Milk is important in a child's diet.*

dieta f. (ethn.) *40 days following parturi-*
tion, puerperium. No se permite dormir
con el esposo durante la dieta. *It is not*
permitted to sleep with one's husband
during the dieta. (Syn: cuarentena)

dificultad f. *difficulty, trouble.* Tiene
dificultades porque no se adapta bien a
las circunstancias. *He has difficulties*
because he doesn't adapt well to the
circumstances.

dificultad al tragar *difficulty in swallowing,*
dysphagia. Un dolor de la garganta causa
dificultad al tragar. *A sore throat makes*
it hard to swallow.

dificultad al respirar *shortness of breath,*
dyspnea. Cuando subí la escalera, tuve
dificultad al respirar. *When I climbed*
the stairs I was short of breath. (Syn:
corto de respiración)

difteria f. *diphtheria.* La difteria afecta la
garganta. *Diphtheria affects the throat.*

digestión f. *digestion.* Se dice que el vino
ayuda a la digestión. *It is said that wine*
helps digestion.

disentería f. *dysentery, diarrhea with*
blood. Varias enfermedades intestinales
están caracterizadas por disentería. *Vari-*
ous intestinal diseases are characterized
by bloody diarrhea. (Syn: obrar con
sangre)

dislocación f. *dislocation, subluxation.* No se le quebró la muñeca pero sí sufrió una dislocación. *His wrist did not break but he did suffer a dislocation.*

disminuirse v. *to get smaller, diminish.* El tumor se disminuye con el tratamiento de rayo equis. *The tumor got smaller with the x-ray therapy.*

dispepsia f. *indigestion, dyspepsia.* La dispepsia puede referirse a cualquier malestar en el estómago. *"Dyspepsia" may refer to any kind of upset stomach.* (Syns: estómago sucio, indigestión)

doblado, -a adj. *bent.* Acuéstese en el lado izquierdo con la pierna derecha doblada. *Lie down on the left side with the right leg bent.* —v. doblar.

doctor, -a n. *doctor.* Un doctor cura enfermedades. *A doctor cures diseases.* (Syn: médico)

dolencia f. *ache.* He tenido una dolencia en la pierna que me está preocupando. *I've been having an ache in the leg that is worrying me.*

doler v. *to hurt, ache.* Me duele mucho el pecho. *My chest hurts a great deal.*

dolor m. *pain.* Tengo un dolor. *I have a pain.* 1. *Qualitative differences: (a)* punzante *throbbing.* La muela podrida motiva un dolor punzante. *A decayed tooth causes a throbbing pain. (b)* picante *stabbing, sticking.* La picada de la avispa deja un dolor picante. *A wasp bite leaves a sticking pain. (c)* agudo, -a *sharp.* El apendis inflamado da un dolor agudo. *An inflamed appendix gives a sharp pain.* 2. *Quantitative differences: (a)* leve, ligero, -a *light.* El rasguño causa un dolor leve. *A scratch causes a light pain. (b)* fuerte *strong.* Tengo un dolor fuerte donde me operaban. *I have a strong pain where they operated on me. (c)* insistente *persistent.* El dolor insistente no se le va. *His persistent pain won't go away. (d)* recio *intractable.* El cáncer puede motivar un dolor recio. *Cancer can cause an intractable pain.*

dolor de *pain in, disease of. Common examples:* vesícula biliar *gall bladder disease;* cabeza *headache;* oído *earache;* garganta *sore throat;* estómago *stomachache;* muela *toothache.*

dolor al orinar *painful urination, dysuria.* Ya llevo una semana con un dolor al orinar. *For a week I have had painful urination.*

dolor de *illness of, literally pain or ache.* El niño se queja de dolor de estómago. *The child complained of stomachache.*

dolor de bazo (coll.) *stitch in side, spleen pain. Folk concept that pain is located in spleen.* Cuando uno corre demasiado, puede ocurrir un dolor de bazo. *When one runs too much, one can get a stitch in the side.*

dolor de cabeza *headache.* El tumor le causó dolor de cabeza por años. *The tumor caused the headache for years.*

dolor de oído *earache.* El bebé tenía un dolor de oído que le hacía llorar. *The baby had an earache that caused him to cry.*

dolores del parto *labor pains, contractions.* Cuando llegan los dolores del parto es hora de irse al hospital. *When labor pains begin it is time to go to the hospital.*

dormir v. *to sleep.* ¿Cuántas horas durmió Ud. anoche? *How many hours did you sleep last night?*

drenaje m. *drain; catheter.* Le pusieron drenaje en el abdomen después de operarla. *They placed a catheter in the abdomen after operating on her.*

droga f. *drug.* La morfina es una droga que se usa medicinalmente. *Morphine is a drug that is used medicinally.*

drogadicto, -a n. *drug addict.* Los drogadictos no pueden funcionar como entes sociales. *Drug addicts cannot function as social beings.*

E

echado a perder *spoiled.* La criatura estaba echada a perder porque le prestaban atención sólo cuando era traviesa. *The child was spoiled because they only paid attention to him when he was mischievous.* (Syns: mimado, chípili)

echar dientes *to teethe.* Los bebés suelen llorar cuando echan dientes. *Babies often cry when they are teething.*

embarazada adj. *pregnant.* Salió embarazada porque no tomaba la píldora como debía. *She got pregnant because she wasn't taking the pill as she should.* (Syns: encinta, gorda, con familia)

embarazo m. *pregnancy.* No le dieron dificultades ni el embarazo ni el parto. *Neither the pregnancy nor the birth gave her any difficulty.*

embolio m. (var. of embolia) *stroke.* Lo que llaman embolio es realmente derrame del cerebro. *What is called* embolio *is really a cerebral hemorrhage.* (Syns: estroc, derrame cerebral)

emborracharse v. *to get drunk.* Unos hombres se ponen violentos cuando se emborrachan. *Some men get violent when they get drunk.*

emoción f. *emotion.* No puede controlar sus emociones: está enojado. *He cannot control his emotions: he is angry.*

empacho m. *constipation.* Le dieron un laxante al niño cuando tuvo un empacho. *They gave a laxative to the child when he had constipation.*

empacho m. (ethn.) *digestive dysfunction. Ethnomedical condition caused by the adherence of undigested food in some part of the gastrointestinal tract. Ritual treatment lasting 3 or 9 days includes massage of back and legs, administration of* añil. Se le pega algo de la comida en los intestinos cuando tiene empacho. *Food sticks in the intestines when one has* empacho.

empeine m. *instep; groin.* El zapato apretado me lastima el empeine. *The tight shoe hurts my instep.*

empeorarse v. *to get worse.* Se empeoró porque la medicina no tuvo ningún efecto. *He got worse because the medicine had no effect.* (Syn: agravarse)

empujar v. *to push.* "Empuje," dijo la partera para que la madre ayudara al parto. *"Push," said the midwife so that the mother would help the delivery.*

en ayunas *while fasting, on an empty stomach.* Hay que tomar ciertas medicinas en ayunas. *Some medicines must be taken on an empty stomach.*

encía f. *gum, gingiva.* Si las encías se infectan, pueden perderse los dientes. *If the gums get infected, one can lose one's teeth.*

encinta adj. (estar) *pregnant.* See **embarazada.**

enchinarse la piel *to get goose bumps or goose flesh.* Se me enchinó la piel cuando salí de la casa al aire frío. *I got goose bumps when I went out in the cold air.* (Syn: ponerse chinito)

enderezar v. *to straighten or to reduce (fracture).* Es preciso enderezar un hueso roto antes de enyesarlo. *It's necessary to straighten a broken bone before putting a cast on it.*

endurecimiento m. *lump, induration.* Un endurecimiento indica que la prueba de piel es positiva. *An induration indicates a positive skin test.* (Syn: bolita)

enema m. *enema.* Le dieron un enema como purgante en el hospital. *They gave him an enema as a purgative at the hospital.* (Syn: lavativa)

enferma adj. *euphemism for menstruating.* La abuela cree que la señorita no debe nadar cuando esta 'enferma.' *The Grandmother believes that young ladies should not swim when they menstruate.*

enfermarse v. *to get sick.* El obrero se enfermó porque no se cuidaba. *The worker got sick because he didn't take care of himself.*

enfermedad benigna *mild disorder, ailment.* Aunque es una enfermedad benigna, hay que tratarla para evitar que se vuelva crónica. *Even though it is a mild disorder, it must be treated to prevent its becoming chronic.*

enfermedad cardíaca *cardiac disease.* La enfermedad cardíaca le causó la debilidad. *The cardiac disease caused his weakness.*

enfermedad congénita *congenital disease.* La sífilis puede ser una enfermedad congénita. *Syphilis can be a congenital disease.*

enfermedad contagiosa *communicable disease.* La viruela loca es una enfermedad muy contagiosa. *Chicken pox is a very contagious disease.*

enfermedad corporal *physical disease.* Normalmente los psiquiatras no curan enfermedades corporales. *Normally psychiatrists do not cure physical diseases.* (Syns: enfermedad física, enfermedad del cuerpo)

enfermedad crónica *chronic disease.* Las enfermedades crónicas son las que duran mucho tiempo. *Chronic diseases are those which last a long time.*

enfermedad de *disease of. Many diseases are named by the organ that is attacked.* La enfermedad del corazón mata a mucha gente. *Heart disease kills many people.* (Syn: mal de)

enfermedad de andancia *disease that's "going around."* La gripe es una de las enfermedades de andancia del invierno. *Flu is one of the diseases that goes around in the winter.* (Syn: enfermedad que anda)

enfermedad del carácter *disease of social pathology, character disorder.* Los criminales padecen de enfermedades de carácter. *Criminals suffer from diseases of social pathology.* (Syn: enfermedad moral)

enfermedad del cuerpo *physical disease.* See **enfermedad corporal.**

enfermedad endañada *disease resulting from acts of witchcraft, hex, spell.* La hechicería es la causa de las enfermedades endañadas. *Witchcraft is the cause of diseases resulting from hexes.*

enfermedad física *physical disease.* See **enfermedad corporal.**

enfermedad grave *serious disease.* El cáncer es una enfermedad grave. *Cancer is a serious disease.*

enfermedad hereditaria *inherited disease, hereditary disease.* La hemofilia es una enfermedad hereditaria. *Hemophilia is a hereditary disease.* (Syn: herencia)

enfermedad mental *mental disease or disturbance.* Necesita un psiquiatra porque padece de una enfermedad mental. *He needs a psychiatrist because he is suffering from a mental disorder.* (Syn: enfermedad emocional)

enfermedad moral *character disorder, disease of social pathology.* La cleptomanía es una enfermedad moral. *Kleptomania is a character disorder.* (Syn: enfermedad del carácter)

enfermedad pasajera *temporary* or *self-limited disease.* La mayoría de las enfermedades pasajeras son las que pegan a los niños. *Most of the self-limited diseases are those which attack children.* (Syn: enfermedad temporal)

enfermedad que anda *disease "that's going around."* See **enfermedad de andancia.**

enfermedad secreta *venereal disease.* Las enfermedades secretas pueden resultar de las relaciones sexuales. *Venereal diseases can come from sexual relations.* (Syn: enfermedad venérea)

enfermedad temporal *temporary or passing disease.* See **enfermedad pasajera.**

enfermedad venérea *venereal disease.* See **enfermedad secreta.**

enfermera, -o n. *nurse.* La enfermera estudia para su profesión en la universidad. *The nurse studies for her profession at the university.*

enfermo, -a n. *sick person.* El enfermo no quiere comer. *The sick person does not want to eat.*

enfocar la vista *to focus.* Después del accidente no pudo enfocar la vista. *After the accident he could not focus.*

engrandecerse v. *to get larger.* El dedo infectado se engrandecía más cada día. *The infected finger got bigger every day.* (Syn: hacerse más grande)

engendrar v. *to engender, procreate, beget.* Después de la vasectomía no podía engendrar hijos. *After his vasectomy he couldn't beget children.* (Syn: procrear)

enjuagar v. *to rinse.* "Enjuague la boca," dice el dentista. *"Rinse your mouth," says the dentist.*

enmohecerse v. *to mold, mildew.* Si el queso se deja al aire se enmohece. *If cheese is left out, it molds.*

enojarse v. *to get angry.* El enojarse sin causa puede ser síntoma de enfermedades mentales. *Getting angry for no reason can be a symptom of mental illness.*

enrojecerse v. *to blush.* Se enrojeció porque la situación era indiscreta. *She blushed because the situation was indiscreet.* (Syn: ruborizarse)

enrojecimiento m. *redness.* La fiebre del heno causa enrojecimiento de los ojos. *Hay fever causes red eyes.*

entablillar v. *to splint.* Se entablilló la pierna para evitar que se moviera. *The leg was splinted to prevent movement.* —n. entabilla.

entablazón f. (ethn.) *obstruction, obstipation, severe constipation.* Cuando pasan muchos días sin obrar puede ser porque uno tiene entablazón. *When one has not moved one's bowels for many days it can be intestinal obstruction.*

entrañas f. pl. *entrails, insides, guts.* El niño se queja de que le duelen las entrañas. *The child is complaining that his insides hurt.*

entrarle calores *to get chills.* Le entraron calores cuando tuvo la gripa. *She had chills when she had the flu.*

entuertos m. pl. *afterpains.* Los entuertos son comunes después del nacimiento del segundo hijo. *Afterpains are common after the birth of the second child.*

envenenar v. *to poison.* El arsénico puede envenenar a una persona. *Arsenic can poison a person.*

envidia f. *envy.* La envidia es una enfermedad moral. *Envy is a character disorder.*

envidia f. (ethn.) *envy. Ethnomedical condition characterized by progressive wasting, caused by envy of others projected onto the patient. Rare today.*

epazote m. (herb) *wormseed (Chenopodium ambrosioides). Prepared as a tea and used to treat stomachache, or as vermifuge.*

epidemia f. *epidemic.* Se dice epidemia cuando muchos padecen de la misma enfermedad. *An epidemic is when many suffer from the same disease.*

epilepsia f. *epilepsy, idiopathic epilepsy.* La epilepsia se puede controlar con medicina. *Epilepsy can be controlled with medicine.*

equilibrio m. *balance, equilibrium.* El niño perdió el equilibrio y se cayó. *The child lost his balance and fell down.* (Syn: balance)

erisipela f. (also **dicipela**) *erysipelas.* La erisipela es una infección de la piel y de los tejidos debajo de la piel. *Erysipelas is an infection of the skin and subcutaneous tissue.*

eructar v. *to belch, burp.* Eructó porque comió muy rápido. *He belched because he ate fast.* (Syns: erutar, repetir)

erutar v. *to belch, burp.* See **eructar.**

escalofríos m. pl. *chills.* Los escalofríos son un síntoma del paludismo. *Chills are a symptom of malaria.*

escamoso, -a adj. *rough.* La piel escamosa puede ser una condición heredada. *A rough skin can be an inherited condition.*

escápula f. *shoulder blade, scapula.* El dolor en la escápula derecha puede ser el resultado de una condición de la vesícula biliar. *Pain in the right shoulder blade may be because of a gall bladder condition.*

esconderse v. *to hide oneself.* El paciente se escondió cuando entró el psiquiatra. *The patient hid when the psychiatrist came in.*

escorpión m. *scorpion.* No todos los escorpiones son venenosos. *Not all scorpions are poisonous.* (Syn: alacrán)

escozor m. *smarting sensation, sting.* Sintió escozor cuando pusieron alcohol en la herida. *He felt a sting when they put alcohol on the wound.*

escroto m. *scrotum.* Le picaba el escroto porque tenía tiña. *His scrotum itched because he had a fungus infection.*

escuchar v. *to listen.* El doctor escucha el latido del corazón con un estetoscopio. *The doctor listens to the heartbeat with a stethoscope.*

escupir v. *to spit, to cough up.* Escupe sangre porque padece de tuberculosis. *He is spitting up blood because he is suffering from tuberculosis.*

escurrir las narices *to have a runny nose.* Cuando un catarro empieza las narices se escurren mucho. *When a cold starts, one's nose runs a lot.*

esófago m. *esophagus, gullet.* La comida pasa por el esófago para llegar al estómago. *Food goes through the esophagus to get to the stomach.* (Syn: boca del estómago)

espalda f. *back, shoulders.* Le duele la espalda por levantar tantas cosas pesadas. *His back hurts from lifting so many heavy things.*

especialista m. & f. *specialist.* El ortopédico es especialista en enfermedades de los huesos y de las coyunturas. *An orthopedist is a specialist in diseases of the bones and joints.*

esperma f. *sperm.* La espuma anticonceptiva mata las espermas. *Contraceptive foam kills the sperm.* (Syn: germen)

espeso, -a adj. *thick.* Tiene el cabello espeso. *He has thick hair.*

espina f. *sticker or thorn; fish bone.* Se le clavó una espina en el pie porque andaba descalzo. *A thorn got stuck in his foot because he was walking barefoot.* (Syn: alguate)

espina dorsal *spine, vertebral column.* El viejo tiene una espina muy curva. *The old man has a very curved spine.* (Syn: espinazo)

espinazo m. *spine, vertebral column.* See **espina dorsal.**

espinilla f. *blackhead, comedon.* La adolescente va al dermatólogo porque tiene muchas espinillas. *The adolescent is going to the dermatologist because she has a lot of blackheads.*

espuma f. *foam.* La espuma anticonceptiva es un método de cuidarse. *Foam is a contraceptive method.*

esputo m. *sputum.* Para dar una muestra de esputo, tosa Ud. muy hondo. *To give a sample of sputum, cough deeply.* (Syn: gargajo)

esqueleto m. *skeleton.* El esqueleto se compone de todos los huesos del cuerpo. *The skeleton is composed of all the bones of the body.*

estafiate m. *wormwood (Artemesia mexicana). Prepared as a tea and used in treatment of colic.*

estar a gusto *to be pleased or comfortable.* No está a gusto a causa del ambiente del hospital. *He is not comfortable because of the hospital's atmosphere.*

estar con familia (coll.) *to be pregnant.* See **embarazada.** (Syns: encinta, gorda)

estar con el esposo (la esposa) *euphemism for sexual intercourse.* Algunas mujeres creen que es repugnante estar con el esposo durante la regla. *Some women think it repugnant to have sexual intercourse during the menstrual period.*

estar crudo, -a *to have a hangover.* Después de emborracharme siempre estoy crudo a la manaña siguiente. *I am always hung over the day after getting drunk.*

estar de *to be in.* Nunca sonríe; siempre está de mal humor. *She never smiles; she is always in a bad mood.*

estar desombligado (coll.) *to have an umbilical hernia.* El niño estaba desombligado porque los músculos del vientre todavía no estaban desarrollados. *The child had an umbilical hernia because the muscles of the belly had not yet developed.*

estéril adj. *sterile.* Es estéril porque ha tenido una vasectomía. *He is sterile because he has had a vasectomy.*

esternón m. *sternum, breast bone.* La criatura respiraba tan fuerte que se le encogía el pecho arriba y debajo del esternón. *The baby breathed with such effort that the chest retracted above and below the sternum.* (Syn: hueso del pecho)

estómago m. *stomach.* El estómago es el primer órgano de digestión. *The stomach is the first digestive organ.* (Syn: abdomen)

estómago revuelto *upset stomach.* Tengo revuelto el estómago porque estoy nerviosa. *I have an upset stomach because I am nervous.*

estómago sucio m. *indigestion, dyspepsia.* Tiene el estómago sucio porque comió demasiado. *He has indigestion because he ate too much.* (Syns: dispepsia, indigestión)

estornudar v. *to sneeze.* Estornudó porque había mucho polen en el aire. *She sneezed because there was a lot of pollen in the air.*

estreñido -a adj. *constipated.* El bebé estaba estreñido porque se había deshidratado. *The baby was constipated because he became dehydrated.*

estreñimiento m. *constipation.* Toma un laxante porque padece de estreñimiento. *He takes a laxative because he is suffering from constipation.*

estroc m. *stroke.* La hemorragia en el cerebro le produjo un estroc. *The brain hemorrhage cause his stroke.* (Syns: embolio, derrame cerebral)

examen m. *laboratory examination, lab test.* Le sacaron sangre para hacer un examen de los glóbulos rojos. *They took a blood sample from him to do an examination of the red blood cells.* (Syn: prueba)

examinación f. *examination.* Es buena idea tener una examinación médica cada año. *It is a good idea to have a medical examination each year.*

excremento m. *stool, excrement.* El excremento duro puede causar estreñimiento. *A hard stool may cause constipation.* (Syn: caca)

excremento aguado *mushy stool.* El excremento aguado es síntoma de enfermedad en el niño. *A mushy stool is a sign of illness in the child.* (Syn: caca aguada)

excremento con babas *stool with mucus.* Si los intestinos están infectados uno tiene excremento con babas. *If one's intestines are infected, one has a stool with mucus.* (Syns: excremento con mocosidad, excremento con moco)

excremento con moco *stool with mucus.* See **excremento con babas.**

excremento con mocosidad *stool with mucus.* See **excremento con babas.**

excremento suelto *diarrhea, loose bowels.* Los microbios en el agua le causaron excremento suelto. *Bacteria in the water gave him diarrhea.* (Syns: diarrea, soltura)

excusado m. *toilet.* El niño pidió ir al excusado para orinar. *The child asked to go to the toilet to urinate.*

F

faja f. *binder, girdle.* Antes, las madres llevaban una faja de manta después del parto. *Formerly, mothers wore a binder of heavy cloth after childbirth.*

fajita f. *belly band.* Hoy día las criaturas no llevan fajitas. *Nowadays, babies don't wear belly bands.*

falo m. *phallus.* Unos psiquiatras interpretan los objetos alargados como símbolos del falo. *Some psychiatrists interpret long objects as phallic symbols.*

falsear v. *to sprain.* Se cayó en la calle y se falseó el tobillo. *He fell in the street and sprained his ankle.* (Syn: torcer)

falseo m. *sprain.* Vendaron su tobillo porque había sufrido un falseo. *They bandaged his ankle because he had suffered a sprain.* (Syn: torcedura, dislocación)

faltar v. *to lack.* Me falta el dinero para pagar al médico. *I lack the money to pay the doctor.*

fallar v. *to fail, give out.* Le tenían que trasplantar un riñón porque el suyo le había fallado. *They had to give him a kidney transplant because his gave out.*

fallecer v. *to die, pass away.* Es huérfano porque fallecieron sus padres. *He is an orphan because his parents died.* (Syns: morir)

farmacia f. *drugstore, pharmacy.* Las farmacias venden drogas. *Pharmacies sell drugs.* (Syn: botica)

fatiga f. *fatigue, tiredness.* Sufre fatiga porque hace dos días que no duerme. *He is suffering from fatigue because he has not slept for two days.* (Syn: cansancio)

feliz adj. *happy.* Uno no puede ser feliz siempre. *One cannot always be happy.* (Syn: alegre)

fenómeno m. (coll.) *monstrosity.* La pastilla anticonceptiva no puede causar fenómenos. *The contraceptive pill cannot cause monstrosities.*

feto m. *fetus.* El feto es una criatura que todavía no ha nacido. *The fetus is a baby that has not yet been born.*

fiebre f. *fever.* El niño tiene mucha fiebre; su temperature está a 40°c. *The child has a high fever; her temperature is 40° C.* (Syn: calentura)

fiebre del heno *hay fever.* El polvo en el aire puede causar fiebre del heno. *Dust in the air can cause hay fever.* (Syn: jey fiver)

fiebre del valle *valley fever, coccidiodomycosis.* Si uno tiene fiebre del valle, uno siempre está fatigado. *If one has valley fever, one is always fatigued.*

fiebre reumática rheumatic fever. La fiebre reumática puede afectar el corazón. *Rheumatic fever can affect the heart.*

fiebre tifoidea *typhoid fever.* La calentura llega a ser muy alta en la fiebre tifoidea. *The temperature becomes very high during typhoid fever.*

flaco, -a adj. *skinny.* Es flaca; no es gorda. *She is skinny; she is not fat.*

flaqueza f. *skinniness.* La flaqueza puede ser mala. *Thinness can be bad.*

flema f. *mucus, phlegm.* El niño tenía mucha flema a causa de la infección pulmonar. *The child had a lot of mucus because of his pulmonary infection.* (Syn: mocosidad)

flujo m. *discharge (old term seldom used today).* El color del flujo puede indicar el tipo de infección. *The color of the discharge can indicate the kind of infection.* (Syn: desecho)

fracasar v. *to fail.* Fracasó como padre porque no se interesaba en sus hijos. *He failed as a father because he didn't take an interest in his children.*

fracturar v. *to break, fracture.* Suele ocurrir que los niños fracturan una pierna. *It often happens that children break a leg.* (Syn: quebrar)

fregar v. *to scrub.* Los trastes deben de fregarse con agua muy caliente y con jabón. *Dishes should be scrubbed with hot water and soap.*

frente f. *forehead.* Tenía sudor en la frente porque hacía calor. *There was sweat on his forehead because it was hot out.*

fresco, -a adj. *cool.* En el verano hace más fresco bajo los árboles. *It is cooler under the trees in the summer.*

fresco, -a adj. *fresh.* Es muy nutritiva la fruta fresca. *Fresh fruit is very nutritious.*

frío, -a *cold.* Las bebidas frías son buenas para los enfermos con calentura. *Cold drinks are good for sick people with fever.*

frío de la matriz (ethn.) *literally cold womb, frigidity, lack of sexual desire. By extension, sterility.* Ella no quiere estar con el esposo a causa del frío de la matriz. *She does not want to have intercourse with her husband because she is frigid.*

frotar v. *to rub.* Le frotaron la frente con alcohol despúes del desmayo. *They rubbed his forehead with alcohol after the fainting spell.*

fuera de prep. *outside of.* Cuando el hombre acaba fuera de la esposa (en el acto sexual) dicen que cuida a la esposa. *When the husband practices withdrawal in sexual intercourse, they say he is "taking care of his wife."*

fuerte adj. *strong.* Cuando esté Ud. más fuerte, puede levantar cosas mas pesadas. *When you are stronger, you can lift heavier things.*

fuertemente *tightly.* Apriete la mano fuertemente. *Close your hand tightly.*

fuerza f. *strength.* La enfermedad le quitó la fuerza. *The illness took away his strength.*

fumar v. *to smoke.* Es peligroso fumar tabaco. *It is dangerous to smoke tobacco.*

G

ganas de comer *appetite.* El no tiene ganas de comer. *He has no appetite.* (Syn: apetito)

gangrena f. *gangrene.* Una infección se puede convertir en gangrena en los diabéticos. *An infection can become gangrene in diabetics.*

gargajo m. *mucus, sputum.* El tísico arroja gargajos de los pulmones. *The tuberculous patient spits mucus from the lungs.* (Syn: esputo)

garganta f. *throat.* Se le ve roja la garganta cuando está inflamada. *The throat looks red when it is inflamed.*

garrapata f. *tick.* Hay que sacar las garrapatas con fuego cuando ya están prendidas. *Once they are attached, ticks must be removed with fire.*

gas m. *gas, flatus.* Los frijoles le dan gas. *Beans give him gas.* (Syns: viento, aire, pedo)

gasa f. *gauze.* La llaga que drena mucha pus puede estar cubierta con una gasa. *A sore that has a lot of pus may be covered with gauze.*

gatear v. *to crawl.* Muchas criaturas aprenden a gatear antes de caminar. *Many babies learn how to crawl before walking.*

gaznate m. (coll.) *windpipe, trachea.* Se la había atorado un pedazo de hielo en el gaznate. *A piece of ice had gotten stuck in the windpipe.*

gelatina anticonceptiva f. *contraceptive jelly.* La gelatina anticonceptiva mata a las espermas. *Contraceptive jelly kills the sperm.*

gemelo -a n. *twin.* Los gemelos idénticos son del mismo óvulo. *Identical twins develop from the same ovum.* (Syn: cuate)

germen m. *sperm.* La espuma anticonceptiva mata el germen. *Contraceptive foam kills the sperm.* (Syn: esperma)

giba f. *hump.* No podía pararse derecho porque tenía una giba. *He couldn't stand up straight because he had a hump.* (Syns: joroba, joma)

ginecólogo, -a n. *gynecologist.* Las mujeres deben consultar a un ginecólogo antes de casarse. *Women should consult a gynecologist before marrying.*

glándula f. *gland.* Las glándulas parótidas se hinchan si uno tiene paperas. *Parotid glands swell up if one has mumps.*

golpe m. *blow; bump.* Salió del accidente sin un golpe. *He came out of the accident without a bump.*

golondrina f. *spurge (Euphorbia maculata).*
Prepared as a tea and used to treat
diarrhea. Also prepared as a solution and
applied to sores and warts.

golpear v. *to strike, hit.* Los padres golpea-
ban al niño cuando se sentían frustrados.
The parents would strike the child when
they felt frustrated. (Syn: pegar)

golpearse v. *to hurt oneself, usually by a*
blow. Se golpeó con el techo bajo. *He*
hurt himself on the low roof.

gómito m. (phonetic variation of **vómito**)
vomit.

gonorrea f. *gonorrhea, clap.* La gonorrea es
una enfermedad venérea. *Gonorrhea is a*
venereal disease. (Syns: purgación,
chorro)

gorda adj. *euphemism for pregnant.*
Cuando una está gorda a veces le
molesta el humo de los cigarros. *When*
one is pregnant, sometimes she is
bothered by cigarette smoke. (Syns:
embarazada, encinta, con familia)

gordo, -a adj. *fat, plump.* Un hombre gordo
usa calzones grandes. *A fat man uses*
large trousers.

gordura f. *fatness, obesity.* La gordura no
es saludable. *Obesity is not healthy.*

gota f. *drop.* Muchas medicinas se miden
por gotas. *Many medicines are measured*
by drops.

gota f. *gout.* La gota es un tipo de artritis
más común en el hombre que en la
mujer. *Gout is a type of arthritis more
common in men than in women.*

gotas de polio *polio drops, oral vaccine.* Se
puede prevenir la poliomielitis dando
gotas de polio por la boca. *Poliomyelitis
may be prevented by oral polio drops.*

gotear v. *to drip.* El suero tiene que gotear
despacio en las venas. *The solution must
drip slowly into the veins.*

gotero m. *eye dropper.* Es bueno usar el
gotero para poner medicina en los ojos.
*It is good to use an eye dropper to put
medicine in the eyes.*

granada f. (herb) *pomegranate (Punica
granatum). Prepared as a tea and used to
treat colic. A solution can also be
gargled for treatment of tonsilitis.*

grano m. *pimple, general skin lesion.* Los
adolescentes tienden a tener granos.
Adolescents tend to have pimples.

grano en el ojo *sty, hordeolum.* Cuando está
irritado el párpado, puede salir un grano
en el ojo. *When the eyelid is irritated, a
sty may come out.* (Syn: perilla en el
ojo)

grano enterrado *boil, furuncle.* Solamente
los médicos pueden tratar los granos
enterrados. *Only doctors can treat boils.*

gratis adv. *free.* Le dan a uno la pastilla gratis en el centro de salud. *They give the pill free at the health department.*

grieta f. *crack, fissure.* La humedad puede causar grietas en las tetillas. *Dampness can cause cracks in the nipples.*

gripe f. (also gripa) *grippe, flu.* Muchos se enferman con la gripe en el invierno. *Many people get sick with the flu in winter.*

gusano m. *worm, parasite.* Los gusanos salen del recto de la niña durante de la noche. *The worms come out of the rectum of the child at night.* (Syn: lombriz)

gustarle a uno *to like.* La berenjena no le gusta a mi niño de dos años. *My two-year-old boy doesn't like eggplant.*

H

hábito m. *habit; religious habit.* Lleva el hábito de San Francisco porque le hizo una manda. *He wears the habit of St. Francis because he made a vow to him. (A vow may be made to wear the habit of a specific saint if he intercedes for a cure.)*

hablar v. *to speak.* Normalmente los niños empiezan a hablar en su segundo año. *Normally children begin speaking in the second year.*

hacer buche *to puff out.* Haga buche con la boca. *Puff out your cheeks.*

hacer caca *to move the bowels.* Al cumplir los dos años, el niño empezó a hacer caca en el excusado. *Upon reaching two years, the child began to move his bowels in the toilet.* (Syn: obrar)

hacer gárgaras *to gargle.* Use agua caliente con sal para hacer gárgaras. *Gargle with hot salt water.*

hacer provecho *to be beneficial.* ¡Ojalá que esta medicina le haga provecho! *I hope this medicine benefits you.*

hacer daño *to damage, harm.* La medicina que tomó la señora le hizo daño. *The medicine the lady took harmed her.*

hacerse daño *to injure or hurt oneself.* No se hizo daño el niño cuando se cayó de la escalera. *The child did not hurt himself when he fell from the stairs.* (Syn: lastimarse)

hacerse más grande *to get larger.* El tumor se hace más grande. *The tumor is getting larger.* (Syn: engrandecerse)

hambre f. (el) *hunger.* El hambre es un problema en los países subdesarrollados. *Hunger is a problem in underdeveloped countries.*

hechicería f. *witchcraft, bewitchment.* Poca gente cree en la hechicería hoy en día. *Few people believe in witchcraft nowadays.*

hechicero, -a n. *sorcerer.* Los hechiceros practican la magia negra. *Sorcerers practice black magic.*

heder v. (coll.) *to stink.* El mal aliento puede heder mucho. *Bad breath can really stink.* (Syn: apestar)

hediondez f. *stench.* See **hedor.**

hedor m. *stench.* No pudo soportar el hedor del mal aliento. *She could not stand the stench of bad breath.* (Syn: hediondez)

hemorragia f. *hemorrhage.* El aborto provocado puede causar hemorragia. *An induced abortion may cause hemorrhage.* (Syn: sangramiento)

hepatitis f. *hepatitis.* Una clase de hepatitis es causada por una virus transmitida por el agua. *One kind of hepatitis is caused by a virus that is transmitted in the water.*

herencia f. (coll.) *inheritance; hereditary disease.* La tuberculosis es una enfermedad contagiosa, no es una herencia. *Tuberculosis is a communicable disease, not a hereditary disease.* (Syn: enfermedad hereditaria)

herida f. *hurt, injury, wound.* Una herida limpia no se infecta. *A clean wound does not get infected.* (Syns: lastimadura, coco)

hernia f. *hernia.* Cuando le resalta a uno una víscera, esto se llama una hernia. *When one's viscera get out of place, it is called a hernia.* (Syn: rotura)

hervir v. *to boil.* El hervir el agua mata a ciertos microbios. *The boiling of water kills some germs.*

hierba f. (also **yerba**) *herb.* Los remedios caseros a veces consisten en hierbas. *Household remedies sometimes consist of herbs.*

hierba colorada (herb) *dock (Rumex crispus). Prepared as a solution and gargled in treatment of tonsilitis.*

hierba del burro (herb) *burro bush (Hymenoclea sp.). Prepared as a solution and applied to arthritic areas and infected cuts.*

hierba del indio (herb) *desert milkweed (Asclepias sp.). Prepared as a tea and used to treat kidney ailments.*

hierba del manzo (herb) *swamp root (Anemopsis californica). Prepared as a tea and used to treat stomachache.*

hierba del pasmo (herb) *spasm herb (Haplopappus larincofolius).* *Prepared as a tea and either drunk or inhaled in the treatment of* pasmo.

hierros m. pl. *forceps.* Sacaron a la criatura con hierros. *The baby was delivered with forceps.* (Syn: pinzas)

hígado m. *liver.* La hepatitis es una enfermedad del hígado. *Hepatitis is a disease of the liver.*

higiene f. *hygiene.* La buena higiene es muy importante para la salud. *Good hygiene is very important for health.*

hilo m. *thread.* El hilo del *coil* debe revisarse por lo menos una vez al mes. *The thread from the coil should be checked at least once a month.*

hincarse v. *to kneel.* Le dolieron las rodillas de tanto hincarse. *Her knees hurt from kneeling so much.*

hincharse v. *to swell.* Las partes dañadas se hinchan. *Injured parts swell.*

hinchazón f. *swelling.* Una compresa fría alivió la hinchazón. *A cold compress reduced the swelling.*

hipo m. *hiccups.* A veces las sodas le dan a uno hipo. *Sometimes soda pop gives one hiccups.*

histeria f. *hysteria.* Las personas con histeria lloran y gritan. *Hysterical persons cry and shout.*

hombro m. *shoulder.* El jugador de fútbol tiene hombros anchos. *The football player has wide shoulders.*

honda para el brazo *sling.* Es necesario usar una honda para un brazo quebrado. *It is necessary to use a sling on a broken arm.*

hongos m. pl. *fungi.* La infección de hongos da mucha comezón. *A fungus infection itches a lot.*

hormigueo m. *prickling pain; tingling sensation, paraesthesia.* Despúes de haber estado sentado por mucho tiempo sentí un hormigueo en los pies. *After sitting so long I had tingling feet.*

hormona f. *hormone.* Las pastillas anticonceptivas están compuestas de hormonas del ovario. *Contraceptive pills are composed of ovarian hormones.*

hoyito m. (del chi o de la orina) *hole, meatus.* El hoyito del chi y el de la vagina son dos aberturas distintas. *The hole for urine and that of the vagina are two different openings.*

hueso m. *bone.* En la niñez los huesos del cuerpo se rompen fácilmente. *In childhood the body's bones break easily.*

hueso del pecho m. *breast bone.* Un dolor agudo debajo del hueso del pecho puede ser señal de un ataque al corazón. *A sharp pain underneath the breast bone may be a sign of a heart attack.* (Syn: esternón)

hueso de la rodilla *knee cap, patella.* El doctor pega debajo del hueso de la rodilla para probar el reflejo. *The doctor taps below the knee to test the reflex.*

huevo m. *egg, ovuum.* El huevo es fertilizado por la esperma. *The egg is fertilized by sperm.* (Syn: óvulo)

huevos m. pl. (coll.) *testicles.* El motociclista dice que ha dañado sus huevos. *The motorcyclist says he has injured his testicles.* (Syn: testículos)

hule m. *condom, prophylactic, rubber.* El hule protege al hombre de una enfermedad venérea. *The rubber protects the man from venereal disease.* (Syns: condón (m.), preservativo)

húmedo, -a adj. *damp.* Los hongos crecen en lugares húmedos. *Fungi grow in humid places.*

humo m. *smoke, smog.* El humo está contaminando el aire del valle. *Smog contaminates the valley air.*

I

incómodo, -a adj. *uncomfortable.* Un dolor de cabeza es incómodo. *A headache is uncomfortable.*

indicar v. *to point to.* Indique la punta de la nariz. *Point to the tip of your nose.*

indigestión f. *indigestion.* Tenía indigestión porque había comido demasiado. *He had indigestion because he had eaten too much.* (Syn: dispepsia, estómago sucio)

infarto del corazón *heart attack, coronary, myocardial infarction.* Un infarto del corazón puede venir del encierro de una arteria del corazón. *A heart attack may be caused by the closing off of a coronary artery.* (Syn: ataque al corazón)

infección f. *infection.* La herida estaba hinchada a causa de la infección. *The wound was swollen on account of the infection.*

infección de la sangre *syphilis.* Se dice infección de la sangre para evitar decir sífilis. *One says "bad blood" to avoid saying syphilis.* (Syns: sifilis, mal de la sangre)

inflamación f. *inflammation.* Las características de una inflamación son calor, dolor, hinchazón y enrojecimiento. *The characteristics of inflammation are heat, pain, swelling, and redness.*

influenza f. *influenza.* La influenza es más grave que un resfriado. *Influenza is more than a simple cold.*

ingle f. *groin, inguinal region.* La comezón de la ingle puede ser causada por piojos o pulgas. *Itching of the groin may be caused by lice or fleas.* (Syn: aldilla)

inmundo, -a adj. *filthy.* La casa de la viejita estaba inmunda. *The little old woman's house was filthy.* (Syn: asqueroso)

inmunización *immunization.* Los niños deben tener inmunizaciones contra la difteria. *Children should have immunizations against diphtheria.* (Syns: inyección contra, vacuna, chot)

inocente adj. *euphemistic reference to various degrees of mental retardation.* El niño inocente no puede asistir a clases regulares. *The retarded child cannot attend regular classes.*

inquieto, -a adj. *restless.* Después de pasar tres días en cama, se puso inquieto. *He became restless after spending three days in bed.*

insolación f. *sunstroke.* Sufrió una insolación por haber estado en el sol por mucho tiempo. *She suffered sunstroke from being in the sun a long time.*

intestino m. *intestine.* No es necesario purgar los intestinos. *It isn't necessary to purge the intestines.* (Syn: tripas)

inválido, -a n. *invalid.* Quedó inválido de la guerra. *He became an invalid as a result of the war.*

inyección f. (contra) *injection, shot, vaccination, immunization.* ¿Ha recibido su niño una inyección contra la difteria? *Has your child received an immunization against diphtheria?* (Syns: vacuna, inmunización, chot)

ir al baño *to go to the bathroom.* Tuvo que ir al baño frecuentemente cuando tenía diarrea. *He had to go to the bathroom frequently when he had diarrhea.*

izquierdo, -a adj. *left.* Quiero examinarle el ojo izquierdo. *I want to examine your left eye.*

J

jadear v. (coll.) *to pant.* Trabajó demasiado fuerte y se puso a jadear. *He worked too hard and began to pant.*

jalar v. *to pull.* Jaló el vaso hacia sí. *He pulled the glass toward himself.*

jalón m. *yank.* Le da un jalón al niño. *He gives a yank to the child.*

jaqueca f. *migraine.* Generalmente se siente la jaqueca en sólo un lado de la cabeza. *Generally a migraine is felt on only one side of the head.*

jarabe m. *(medicinal) syrup.* Hay varios jarabes para la tos. *There are various syrups for cough.*

jey fiver *hay fever.* El polen de la hierba le daba jey fiver. *Grass pollen gave him hay fever.* (Syn: fiebre del heno)

jiricua f. *vitiglio, pie baldness.* Muchos carnales en mi familia tuvieron jiricua. *Many of my blood relatives had vitiglio.*

joma f. *hump.* La vieja tiene una joma en la espalda. *The old lady has a hump on her back.* (Syns: joroba, giba)

joroba f. *hump.* See **joma**.

jorobado, -a adj. *hunch-backed.* El niño nació jorobado. *The child was born hunch-backed.*

juanete m. *bunion.* Después de llevar zapatos apretados por tantos años le salió un juanete. *From wearing tight shoes so many years, a bunion was caused.*

jugar v. *to play.* El jugar ayuda al desarrollo de los niños. *Playing aids children's development.*

juguete m. *toy.* Las muñecas son los juguetes favoritos de las niñas. *Dolls are the favorite toys of girls.*

juntarse v. (coll.) *to have intercourse.* Para alguna gente es pecado juntarse antes de casarse. *For some people it is a sin to have intercourse before marriage.*

K

kilo m. *2.2 pounds.* Al nacer la criatura pesaba tres kilos. *At birth the baby weighed 6.6 pounds.*

L

labio m. *lip.* Se puede evitar los labios rajados usando crema. *Chapped lips may be prevented by using cream.*

labio cucho *harelip.* La luz de la luna no puede causar el labio cucho. *Moonlight cannot cause harelip.* (Syn: labio leporino)

labio leporino *harelip.* See **labio cucho.**

ladilla f. *crab louse (Phthirus pubis).* Un mujeriego puede tener ladillas. *The libertine can have crab lice.*

lágrima f. *tear.* Las lágrimas sirven para limpiar el ojo. *Tears serve to clean the eye.*

lagrimar v. *to tear.* Sus ojos estaban lagrimando a causa de las alergias. *His eyes were tearing because of allergies.*

lamber v. *to lick.* Le gusta lamber paletas. *He likes to lick popcicles.*

lanten m. (herb) *plantain (Plantago mayor). Prepared as a tea and used to treat dysentery. A solution is also gargled for a sore throat.*

laringe f. *larynx.* La voz viene de la laringe. *The voice comes from the larynx.*

lástima f. (tener) *pity (to feel).* Le tenía lástima a la criatura porque estaba deformada. *He felt pity for the baby because it was deformed.*

lastimadura f. *hurt, injury, wound.* Sufrió una lastimadura del muslo cuando se cayó del columpio. *He suffered an injury to his thigh when he fell from the swing.* (Syns: herida, coco)

lastimarse v. *to injure or hurt oneself.* Al caerse de la escalera, se lastimó la niña. *The little girl hurt herself when she fell off the ladder.* (Syn: hacerse daño)

latido m. (ethn.) *gnawing sensation, characterized by notable beating of the abdominal aorta. If not corrected with bland food immediately, may cause discomfort for days. Formerly conceived of as starvation.* Porque el viejo no podía comer, sufrió latido. *Because the old man could not eat he got latido.*

latido m. *heartbeat.* Los latidos del corazón deben ser regulares. *Heartbeats should be regular.* (Syn: lato)

latir v. *to beat (the heart).* Una persona está viva hasta que el corazón deja de latir. *A person is alive until his heart stops beating.* (Syn: palpitar)

lato m. *heartbeat.* See **latido.**

lavado vaginal m. *douche.* El lavado vaginal no es necesario para la salud. *A vaginal douche is not necessary for health.*

lavar v. *to wash.* La enfermera lavó al enfermo. *The nurse bathed the patient.*

lavarse la boca *to brush one's teeth.* Para no tener mal aliento es necesario lavarse la boca diariamente. *To not have bad breath it is necessary to brush one's teeth daily.*

lavativa f. *enema.* Antes de la operación le pusieron una lavativa. *Before the operation they gave her an enema.* (Syn: enema)

laxante m. *laxative.* Tomó un laxante porque hacía cuatro días que no obraba. *He took a laxative because he hadn't moved his bowels for four days.*

leche f. *milk.* La leche es nutritiva para los niños. *Milk is nutritious for children.*

leche de bote *evaporated milk.* La leche de bote debe de mezclarse con agua. *Evaporated milk should be mixed with water.* (Syn: leche evaporada)

leche de vaca *fresh milk.* Hay que mezclar la leche de vaca con agua para dársela a las criaturas. *Fresh milk must be mixed with water to be given to infants.* (Syn: leche fresca)

leche evaporada *evaporated milk.* See **leche de bote.**

leche fresca *fresh milk.* See **leche de vaca.**

lengua f. *tongue.* Por favor, saque la lengua. *Please stick out your tongue.*

lepra f. *leprosy, Hansen's disease.* La lepra es una enfermedad no muy común. *Leprosy is an uncommon disease.*

leucemia f. *leukemia.* En la leucemia se aumentan los glóbulos blancos de la sangre. *With leukemia the number of white corpuscles increases.*

levantar v. *to raise, lift.* Levante los hombros para que yo los oprima. *Lift your shoulders so that I can press against them.*

levantarse v. *to get up.* Un día después de la operación le dejaron levantarse. *One day after the operation they let him get up.*

leve adj. *shallow, light.* Tiene una herida leve en la pierna. *He has a shallow wound on the leg.*

liendre f. *nit.* La medicina Qwell disuelve las liendres. *Qwell dissolves nits.*

limpiar v. *to clean.* Hay que limpiar las heridas para que no se infecten. *It is necessary to clean wounds so they will not become infected.*

líquido m. *liquid.* Hay que tomar muchos líquidos cuando uno tiene diarrea. *It is necessary to drink a lot of liquids when one has diarrhea.*

líquido, -a adj. *liquid.* Algunos medicamentos son líquidos. *Some medications are liquid.*

loco, -a adj. *crazy.* Cuando el hombre se volvió loco, lo mandaron al manicomio. *When the man went crazy they took him to a mental hospital.*

locura f. *craziness.* La medicina causó una locura temporal. *The medicine caused a temporary craziness.*

lombriz f. *worm, earthworm.* Las lombrices causan la anemia y los torzones. *Worms cause anemia and cramps.* (Syn: gusano)

lunar m. *mole, nevus, birthmark.* Unos lunares se ponen cancerosos. *Some moles become cancerous.*

Ll

llaga f. *ulcer, open sore.* Las llagas son heridas abiertas o llenas de pus. *Ulcers are wounds which are open or filled with pus.*

llenar v. *to fill.* El boticario llenó la receta. *The druggist filled the prescription.*

llanto m. *weeping; wailing.* El llanto de los niños le molestó. *The children's weeping annoyed her.*

llorar v. *to cry, weep.* El niño lloró cuando le pegó su mamá. *The child cried when his mother slapped him.*

M

machucar v. *to crush.* El niño se machucó el dedo en el cajón. *The child crushed his finger in the drawer.*

madurar v. *to mature, ripen.* Antes decían que las cataratas tenían que madurar. *They used to say that cataracts had to ripen.*

magulladura f. *bruise, contusion.* La magulladura es azul y negra. *The bruise is blue and black.* (Syn: moretón)

mal, -o, -a adj. *poor, bad, not good.* El chico tuvo mal apetito durante su enfermedad. *The child had a poor appetite during his illness.*

mal de *disease, specified by organ or location.* Tengo mal de riñon. *I have a kidney disease.* (Syn: enfermedad de)

mal de hiel *gall bladder disease, cholycystitis.* El mal de hiel es una enfermedad común en las mujeres mayores. *Gall bladder disease is a common disease in older women.* (Syns: dolor de la vesícula biliar, bilis)

mal de ijar (ethn.) *flank pain (from conditions such as appendicitis or pelvic inflammatory disease).* Lo que llaman mal de ijar es realmente seña de varias enfermedades. *What is called mal de ijar is actually a sign of various illnesses.*

mal de la sangre *euphemism for syphilis.* Se puede contraer mal de la sangre por contacto sexual. *One can contract syphilis through sexual contact.*

mal de ojo *pinkeye, conjunctivitis.* El mal de ojo es causado por microbios. *Pinkeye is caused by germs.*

mal de orín (lay) *urinary disease.* Mal de orín puede ser enfermedad de la vejiga, o aún de los riñones. *Urinary disease can be in the bladder or up to the kidneys.*

mal de pinto *pinta.* El mal de pinto es una enfermedad contagiosa; la jiricua es hereditaria. *Pinta is a contagious disease; vitiglio is inherited.*

mal ojo (ethn.) *evil eye. Ancient idea, found transculturally, of illness caused magically by envy. Healthy child is especially vulnerable to glance of someone who is not allowed to touch him. Cured by ritual.* Cuando no la dejaron cogerlo, la mujer le echó mal ojo al niño. *When she could not hold him, the woman cast the evil eye on the child.*

mal parto *miscarriage, spontaneous abortion.* Después de dos meses de embarazo la mujer sufrió un mal parto. *After two months of pregnancy the woman suffered a miscarriage.* (Syn: aborto natural)

malaria f. *malaria.* La malaria causa más muertes que cualquier otra enfermedad del mundo. *Malaria causes more deaths than any other disease in the world.* (Syn: paludismo)

malestar m. *upset, indisposition, malaise.* Siente un malestar en el estómago. *He feels an upset in his stomach.*

malva f. (herb) *mallow (Malva parviflora). Prepared in solution and used as an enema in treating fever.*

mamadera f. *nursing bottle.* La madre decidió darle la mamadera a su bebé porque ella tenía que trabajar. *The mother decided to give the bottle to her baby because she had to work.* (Syns: biberón, tetera, botella)

mamar v. *to nurse.* El saber mamar es reflejo natural. *Knowing how to suck is a natural reflex.*

mancha f. *spot, stain.* Durante el embarazo muchas mujeres tienen manchas en la piel. *During pregnancy many women get spots on their skin.*

mancha azul *mongolian spot.* Las manchas azules en las nalgas son normales en la niñez. *Mongolian spots on the buttocks are normal in childhood.*

manda f. *offer, vow.* Voy a hacer una manda a San Martín. *I am going to make an offer to St. Martin.*

mandíbula f. *jaw, mandible.* La artritis puede pegar a las coyunturas de la mandíbula. *Arthritis can strike the joints of the mandible.* (Syn: quijada)

manicomio m. *mental institution.* Muchos pacientes salen curados del manicomio. *Many patients leave mental institutions cured.*

mano f. *hand.* Por favor, muéstreme la palma de su mano. *Please show me the palm of your hand.*

manosear v. *handle.* No manosées a la criatura. *Don't handle the baby.*

manteca f. *lard.* Es mala idea poner manteca en las quemaduras. *It is a bad idea to put lard on burns.*

mantener v. *to maintain, support.* Tradicionalmente el hombre ha mantenido a su familia. *Traditionally the man has supported the family.*

manzanilla f. (herb) *camomile (Matricaria chamomilla). Prepared as a tea and used to treat colic and labor pains. This is the most common treatment for colic in children.*

marearse v. *to become nauseated and dizzy.* Cuando vamos a pasear en carro, siempre se marea mi hija. *When we go riding in the car my daughter always gets sick.*

mareos m. pl. *dizziness and nausea.* El niño tuvo mareos quando el carro subió la montaña. *The child got dizzy when the car ascended the mountain.*

mascar v. *to chew.* La carne dura es difícil de mascar. *Tough meat is hard to chew.*

mata f. *plant.* El polen de muchas matas causa alergias. *The pollen of many plants causes allergies.* (Syn: planta)

matriz f. *uterus.* La señora tenía un tumor benigno en la matriz. *The lady had a benign tumor in her uterus.*

mear v. (coll.) *to pee, urinate.* ¡No mees en la cama, hijo! *Don't pee in the bed, son!* (Syn: orinar)

mecedora f. *rocking chair.* La mecedora ayuda a dormir a un bebé. *A rocking chair helps put a baby to sleep.*

mecer v. *to rock.* La madre tuvo que mecer a su niño para dormirle. *The mother had to rock the baby to put it to sleep.*

medicina f. *medicine.* Cuando toma medicina, siga las direcciones. *When you take medicine, follow the instructions.*

medicina de la farmacia *patent medicine.* Lidia Pinkham es medicina de la farmacia para mujer. *Lydia Pinkham is a patent medicine for women.* (Syn: medicina de la botica)

médico, -a n. *doctor.* Necesitamos médicos que se dediquen a prevenir enfermedades. *We need doctors who will dedicate themselves to preventing illness.* (Syn: doctor)

médula del hueso *bone marrow, medulla.* Examinaron la muestra de la médula del hueso para cambios en los glóbulos rojos. *They examined the sample of bone marrow for changes in the red blood cells.*

mejilla f. *cheek.* Unos niños tienen mejillas rosadas. *Some children have pink cheeks.* (Syn: cachete)

mejorarse v. *to improve; to get better.* Ojalá que se mejore rápidamente para que pueda regresar a trabajar. *I hope you get better quickly so that you may return to work.*

memoria f. *memory.* La anciana tenía una memoria excelente. *The old woman had an excellent memory.*

meningitis f. *meningitis.* La meningitis puede ser motivada por varios microbios. *Meningitis may be caused by various microorganisms.*

menudo m. *tripe soup.* El menudo es un caldo de tripas con nixtamal. *Menudo is a soup of tripe with hominy.*

menopausia f. *menopause, change of life.* La menopausia ocurre por lo general después de los cuarenta años. *Menopause generally occurs after forty.* (Syn: cambio de vida)

menstruación f. *menstruation.* La menstruación empieza generalmente a los doce años de edad. *Menstruation generally begins at twelve years of age.* (Syns: periodo, regla)

menstruar v. *to menstruate, to have your period.* La mujer que lleva el coil menstrúa más. *Women with I.U.D.'s menstruate more.* (Syns: estar "enferma," reglar)

mental adj. *mental.* La depresión es una enfermedad mental común. *Depression is a common mental illness.*

mentira f. *lie, falsehood.* Los que dicen muchas mentiras pueden ser casos mentales. *Those who tell a lot of lies may be mental cases.*

merolico m. *quack, charlatan.* El merolico vendió sus curas falsas. *The quack sold his phony cures.* (Syn: charlatán)

mezquino m. *wart.* El chico tenía mezquinos en la mano. *The child had warts on his hand.* (Syn: verruga)

microbio m. *germ, microbe.* Los microbios causan muchas enfermedades. *Germs cause many illnesses.*

miedo m. *fear.* Tiene miedo porque le van a operar. *He is afraid because they are going to operate on him.*

miedoso, -a adj. *fearful.* Fue difícil examinar al chico miedoso. *It was difficult to examine the fearful child.*

milagro m. *miracle.* Parece milagro que ella se sanó. *It seems a miracle that she got well.*

milagro m. (ethn.) *ex voto, effigy. These tiny symbols of cures may be seen on religious statues throughout the Catholic world, where they are called ex votos.* Llevaba un milagro de una pierna a San Francisco porque se le había curado la gangrena. *She carried an effigy of a leg to St. Francis because she was cured of gangrene.*

mimar *to fondle, to indulge.* Es difícil controlar a una criatura que se mima mucho. *It's difficult to control a child that is indulged a lot.*

mirar v. *to look (at).* Mire derecho para que yo pueda examinarle el ojo. *Look straight ahead so I can examine your eye.*

mitad f. *half.* Déle sólo la mitad de la pastilla. *Give him only a half of the pill.*

mocosidad f. *mucus, phlegm.* Está arrojando mocosidades. *He is coughing up mucus.* (Syn: flema, moquera)

mocoso, -a adj. *mucous.* Tiene una úlcera en una membrana mocosa. *He has an ulcer on a mucous membrane.*

mojar v. *to wet.* El bebé mojó la zapeta. *The baby wet the diaper.*

molestia f. *discomfort.* Las puntadas le causan molestia. *The stitches are causing him discomfort.*

mollera f. *soft spot, fontanel (especially anterior).* La mollera se baja con la deshidratación. *The soft spot is depressed with dehydration.*

mollera caída (ethn.) *fallen fontanel; depression of the sagittal or lambdnoidal suture which accompanies dehydration. Ethnic concept that fontanel becomes depressed from a falling of the soft palate. Treatments include pressure on soft palate and suction of fontanel, maintained by egg, salt, or herbs.* Con deshidratación, se puede caer la mollera. *The fontanel can fall from dehydration.*

moquera f. (coll.) *snot, nasal mucus.* Suene la nariz para quitar la moquera. *Blow your nose to get rid of the snot.* (Syns: flema, mocosidad)

morado, -a adj. *purple.* El niño cardiaco tiene los labios morados. *The cardiac child has purple lips.*

morder v. *to bite; clench teeth.* Muerda para que yo pueda examinar la fuerza del nervio. *Bite down so that I may test the strength of the nerve.*

moretón m. *bruise, contusion.* El accidente le dejó muchos moretones por todo el cuerpo. *The accident left him with a lot of bruises all over his body.* (Syn: magulladura)

morir v. *to die, pass away.* El paciente murió en la sala de recuperación. *The patient died in the recovery room.* (Syn: fallecer)

mortificado, -a adj. *worried.* El marido estaba muy mortificado porque iban a operar a su esposa. *The husband was very worried because they were going to operate on his wife.* (Syn: preocupado)

mosca f. *fly.* Las moscas pueden transmitir microbios. *Flies can transmit germs.*

mosquito m. *mosquito; little fly (often applied to small insects).* Los mosquitos se crían en agua estancada. *Mosquitos breed in stagnant water.* (Syn: zancudo)

movimiento m. *movement.* El enfermo no puede controlar los movimientos de los muslos. *The patient cannot control the movements of his thighs.*

muchacho, -a n. *youth (young girl).* Es importante darles valores morales a los muchachos. *It is important to give moral values to children.*

muela f. *molar; any tooth.* Las muelas son los dientes que mastican. *The molars are the teeth that chew.*

muela podrida *decayed molar (tooth in general).* Le sacaron la muela podrida porque era muy dolorosa. *They removed his decayed molar because it was very painful.*

muerte f. *death.* La muerte de sus padres le había afectado al niño. *The death of his parents had affected the child.*

muerto, -a adj. *dead.* Entierran el animal muerto. *They bury the dead animal.*

muestra f. *sample, specimen.* Le tomaron una muestra de orina para ver si estaba embarazada. *They took a urine sample to see if she was pregnant.*

muleta f. *crutch.* Usa una muleta para ayudarle a caminar. *He uses a crutch to help himself walk.*

muñeca f. *wrist.* La artritis pega a los huesos de la muñeca. *Arthritis attacks the bones of the wrist.*

murmullo m. *murmur (abnormal heart sounds).* Algunos murmullos del corazón son inocentes. *Some heart murmurs are harmless.* (Syns: soplo)

músculo m. *muscle.* El ejercicio aumenta el tamaño del músculo. *Exercise increases the size of the muscle.*

muslo m. (var. of murlo) *thigh.* Se dió la inyección en el muslo. *The injection was administered into the thigh.*

N

nacer v. *to be born.* El bebé no pesaba mucho porque nació prematuro. *The baby didn't weigh much because it was born premature.*

nalgas f. pl. *buttocks.* Mueva las nalgas hasta el borde de la mesa, por favor. *Move your buttocks to the edge of the table, please.* (Syn: sentaderas)

naranja f. (herb) *orange leaves (Citrus simenis).* Prepared as a tea and used to treat colic.

narices f. pl. *nostrils.* Respira con dificultad porque tiene las narices constipadas. *He breathes with difficulty because his nostrils are stopped up.*

nariz f. *nose, nostril.* Se chocó contra la puerta y rompió su nariz. *He ran into the door and broke his nose.*

náusea f. *nausea.* Unas mujeres embarazadas sufren de náusea. *Some pregnant women suffer from nausea.*

negrita f. *elderberry (Sambucus mexicana). The berry is prepared as a tea and used to treat colic.*

nervio m. *nerve.* La estricnina es un veneno que ataca los nervios. *Strychnine is a poison that attacks the nerves.*

nervios m. pl. *nervousness.* Ella sufre de nervios. *She suffers from nervousness.*

niña del ojo *pupil (of eye)*. En la oscuridad se engrandece la niña del ojo. *The pupil dialates in the dark.*

niño, -a n. *little boy (little girl), child.* El niño acaba de cumplir cuatro años. *The child has just had his fourth birthday.*

nogal m. (herb) *walnut (Juglans regia).* *Nuts are boiled and the solution is used as a douche to treat hemmorhage.*

nopal m. *prickly pear.* Una ensalada puede llevar nopal, chile verde, tomatillo, perejil, berro y cebolla verde. *Prickly pear, green chile, green tomatoes, parsley, water cress, and green onion may be included in a salad.*

nube del ojo *cataract.* No ve bien porque tiene una nube del ojo. *He doesn't see well because he has a cataract.* (Syn: catarata)

nuca f. *back of the neck.* Le dolía la nuca porque solía leer en la cama. *His neck hurt because he used to read in bed.*

nudillo m. *knuckle.* No puede usar lápiz porque tiene artritis en sus nudillos. *He can't write with a pencil because he has arthritis in his knuckles.*

nudo m. *node; knot.* Después de una infección en la garganta, pueden resultar nudos en el cuello. *After a throat infection nodes may result in the neck.*

nuez de Adán *Adam's apple, thyroid cartilage.* Su nuez de Adán se mueve cuando habla. *His Adam's apple moves when he talks.* (Syn: nuez de la garganta)

nuez de la garganta *Adam's apple, thyroid cartilage.* See **nuez de Adán.**

nutritivo, -a adj. *nutricious.* Algunas comidas son más nutritivas que otras. *Some foods are more nutritious than others.*

O

obrar v. *to move the bowels.* La persona estreñida no puede obrar. *A constipated person cannot move his bowels.* (Syn: hacer caca)

obrar con sangre *to have blood in the stool, dysentery.* Nunca es normal obrar con sangre. *It is never normal to have blood in the stool.* (Syn: disentería)

obstruir v. *obstruct.* Las cataratas de los ojos obstruyen la vista. *Cataracts obstruct vision.* (Syn: atorar)

oftalmólogo, -a n. *ophthalmologist.* Un doctor que examina los ojos es el oftalmólogo. *The ophthalmologist is a doctor who examines eyes.*

oído m. *ear (middle and inner).* No se deben introducir objetos agudos a los oídos. *Sharp objects should not be introduced into the ears.*

oír v. *to hear.* Se puede oír sin escuchar. *One can hear without listening.*

ojo m. *eye.* El color de los ojos es hereditario. *Eye color is inherited.*

ojo de venado (ethn.) *deer's eye (Muzuna sloani). Amulet used for protection against the evil eye.*

oler v. *to smell.* Tiene catarro y no puede oler bien. *She has a cold and cannot smell well.*

olor m. *smell, odor.* Para no caerle mal a la gente es necesario evitar el mal olor personal. *One must avoid bad personal odor in order not to displease others.*

ombligo m. *navel, umbilicus.* Tiene el ombligo salido. *He has a protruding navel.*

oprimir v. *to press against.* El doctor oprime los músculos del paciente para medir la fuerza de él. *The doctor presses against the patient's muscles to measure his strength.*

orégano m. (herb) *oregano (Origanum vulgare). Prepared as a tea and used to bring on a delayed menstrual period as well as in the treatment of a cold.*

oreja f. *ear (external).* Lleva pendientes en las orejas. *She is wearing dangling earrings in her ears.*

órgano m. *organ.* El corazón es un órgano. *The heart is an organ.*

orín m. *urine.* See **orina.**

orina f. *urine.* Ciertas enfermedades causan orina colorada. *Certain illnesses cause reddish urine.* (Syn: orín)

orinar v. *to urinate.* Si uno está tomando mucho orina mucho también. *If one is drinking a lot, one also urinates more.* (Syn: mear)

orinar muy de seguido *urinary frequency.* La gente que sufre de diabetes necesita orinar muy de seguido. *People with diabetes need to urinate frequently.*

orzuelo m. *hordeolum, sty.* Se puede aliviar el orzuelo con ungüentos antibióticos. *A sty can be cured with antibiotic ointment.* (Syns: perilla en el ojo, grano en el ojo)

ovario m. *ovary.* El ovario produce hormonas y óvulos. *The ovary produces hormones and ova.*

óvulo m. *ovuum.* El óvulo es lo que la esperma fertiliza. *The ovuum is what the sperm fertilizes.* (Syn: huevo)

óvulos m. pl. *vaginal suppositories.* Se puede usar óvulos como anticonceptivos. *Vaginal suppositories may be used as contraceptives.*

oxígeno m. *oxygen.* Al que respira con dificultad se le da oxígeno. *Oxygen is given to someone who is having trouble breathing.*

P

paciente m. & f. *patient.* El doctor dio una inyección al paciente. *The doctor gave a shot to the patient.*

padecer de *to suffer from.* Ella padeció de artritis por muchos años. *She suffered from arthritis for many years.* (Syn: sufrir de)

paladar m. *palate.* El paladar es el techo de la boca. *The palate is the roof of the mouth.*

paleta f. *shoulder blade, scapula.* La paleta es parte del hombro. *The scapula is a part of the shoulder.*

palma f. *palm.* Las líneas de la palma no suelen indicar anormalidades. *The lines on the palm do not usually indicate abnormalities.*

palpar v. *to palpate.* El médico puede palpar la hinchazón. *The doctor can palpate the swelling.*

palpitación f. *rapid heart beat, tachycardia.* Cuando uno corre, siente palpitaciones. *When one runs, one notes rapid heart beats.*

palpitar v. *to beat (heart).* El corazón palpita setenta veces por minuto. *The heart beats seventy times a minute.* (Syn: latir)

paludismo m. *malaria; term indiscriminately applied to febrile illness.* Con el paludismo uno sufre de escalofríos y de calenturas. *With malaria one suffers chills and fever.* (Syn: malaria)

pamita f. (herb) *tansy mustard (Descurainia pinnata). Prepared as a tea for the treatment of* empacho.

páncreas m. *pancreas.* El páncreas produce insulina. *The pancreas produces insulin.*

panza f. (coll.) *tummy, belly.* El bebé de tres meses ya tenía una panza gorda. *The three-month-old baby already had a fat tummy.* (Syn: barriga)

panzón, -a adj. *pot-bellied.* Es panzón porque toma mucha cerveza. *He is pot-bellied because he drinks a lot of beer.*

pañal m. *diaper.* Cuesta más usar pañales de papel que pañales de tela. *It costs more to use paper diapers than cloth diapers.* (Syn: zapeta)

paperas f. pl. *mumps.* Las paperas son una infección viral de las glándulas parótidas. *Mumps are an infection of the parotid glands.*

paralizado, -a adj. (estar) *paralized.* Después del estroc el señor estaba paralizado del lado izquierdo. *After the stroke the man was paralyzed on his left side.* —n. parálisis.

pararse v. *to stand up.* El niño de seis meses no se para solo. *The six-month-old child does not stand by himself.* (Syn: ponerse de pie)

parche m. *poultice; plaster.* Un parche de mostaza puede quemar la piel. *A mustard poultice can burn the skin.*

parpadear v. *to blink.* Cuando uno tiene algo en el ojo le hace parpadear. *When one has something in the eye it makes one blink.*

párpado m. *eyelid.* El orzuelo puede causar hinchazón del párpado. *A sty can cause swelling of the eyelid.*

partera f. *midwife (licensed).* Antes era muy común que una partera ayudara al parto. *Previously it was common for midwives to assist in deliveries.*

parte del cuerpo body part. *Para hacer una diagnosis hay que examinar cada parte del cuerpo.* To make a diagnosis, every part of the body must be examined.

partes privadas f. pl. *privates, genitals.* Es importante limpiar las partes privadas de los niños con agua y jabón. *It is important to clean children's privates with soap and water.* (Syn: verijas)

parto m. *delivery, parturition, childbirth, labor.* El parto se llevó a cabo sin novedad. *The delivery was handled without difficulty.*

pasmo m. (ethn.) *infection. Class of diseases caused by changing environmental temperature and characterized by rash and swelling. If precipitated by sun's rays, apply* sauco. *If effected by chilling overheated body, administer* hierba del pasmo. Mi hijo se pasmó porque se bañó cuando tenía fiebre. *My son got* pasmo *when, febrile, he took a bath.*

pasmo del parto *childbed fever.* El pasmo del parto ocurre si hay una infección de microbios. *Childbed fever occurs when there is a bacterial infection.*

pasmo seco (rare) *tetanus, lockjaw.* Si se usan tijeras no esterilizadas en el cordón, puede dar pasmo seco. *If unsterile scissors are used on the umbilical cord, they can confer tetanus.* (Syn: tétano)

pastilla f. *pill; birth control pill.* Las pastillas que me recetó el doctor me hicieron buen provecho. *The pills that the doctor prescribed for me were beneficial.* (Syn: píldora)

pecho m. *chest, thorax.* Sintió un dolor en el pecho a causa de la pleuresía. *He felt a chest pain because of the pleurisy.*

pecho m. *breast.* El doctor le examinó para ver si tenía bolitas en los pechos. *The doctor examined her to see if she had lumps in her breasts.* (Syns: chichi, teta)

pedo m.(coll.) *expelled gas, flatus, fart.* Después de comer frijoles estuvo tirando pedos. *After eating beans he was passing gas.* (Syns: viento, aire)

pegajoso, -a adj. (coll.) *contagious.* La viruela loca es pegajosa. *Chicken pox is contagious.* (Syn: contagioso)

pegar v. *to slap, hit; beat.* Le pegaban al niño cuando no se portaba bien. *They slapped the child when he did not behave well.*

pegarle a uno to catch. Me pegó el sarampión cuando tenía cinco años. *I caught measles when I was five years old.* (Syn: agarrar)

pegarse v. *to cling or stick to.* Las pestañas del niño se pegaron a causa de la pus. *The child's eyelashes stuck together because of the pus.*

pelear v. *to fight.* Los hermanos peleaban mucho cuando eran chicos. *The siblings fought a lot when they were little.*

peligroso, -a adj. *dangerous.* Algunos anti-bióticos pueden ser peligrosos para algunas personas. *Some antibiotics can be dangerous for some people.*

pelo m. *hair.* Algunas jovenes se rasuran el pelo de las piernas. *Some young girls shave the hair on their legs.*

pene m. *penis.* La circuncisión es una operación casi rutina del pene. *Circumcision is an almost routine operation on the penis.*

pensamiento m. *thought.* Cuando empezó a tener pensamientos de suicidio decidió consultar al psiquiatra. *When he began to have thoughts of suicide he decided to consult a psychiatrist.*

pepa f. *clitoris.* La pepa es el sitio de la sensación sexual máxima para la mujer. *The clitoris is the site of highest sexual sensation for the woman.* (Syn: clítoris)

perder v. *to lose.* Durante la enfermedad perdió mucho peso. *During the illness she lost a lot of weight.*

periférico, -a adj. *peripheral.* La vista perifé-rica se disminuye cuando se fuma la marijuana. *Peripheral vision is dimin-ished when marijuana is smoked.*

perilla en el ojo *sty, hordeolum.* Una perilla en el ojo tiene que madurar antes de que se drene. *A sty has to come to a head before it drains.* (Syns: grano en el ojo, orzuelo)

peritonitis f. *peritonitis. Also folk concept that this condition is the result of severe constipation.* Después de que se reventó la apendis le entró peritonitis. *After the appendix burst, peritonitis set in.*

pesadilla f. *nightmare.* La pesadilla despertó al niño. *The nightmare woke up the child.*

pesado, -a adj. *heavy.* Con la ansiedad se siente pesado el pecho. *With anxiety the chest feels heavy.*

pesar v. *to weigh.* Come demasiado y pesa más cada semana. *She eats too much and weighs more every week.*

pescuezo m. (coll.) *neck.* Los dolores del pescuezo a veces son causados por la tensión nerviosa. *Neck pain at times may be caused by nervous tension.*

peso m. *weight.* El bebé aumentaba de peso cada semana. *The baby gained weight each week.*

pestaña f. *eyelash.* Las pestañas ayudan a mantener limpios los ojos. *Eyelashes help keep the eyes clean.*

pezón m. *nipple.* El bebé chupaba el pezón porque tenía hambre. *The baby sucked the nipple because it was hungry.* (Syn: tetilla)

pezón enlechado *engorged nipple, caked breast.* Es necesario exprimir leche para aliviar el pezón enlechado. *It is necessary to express milk in order to alleviate an engorged nipple.*

picada f. *sting.* La picada de la avispa duele mucho. *The wasp's sting hurts a lot.* (Syns: picadura, piquete)

picadura f. *sting, insect bite.* See **picada.**

picar v. *to sting; to bite.* Le picó el zancudo. *The mosquito bit him.*

picar v. *to itch.* La piel le pica al niño porque está seca. *The child's skin itches because it's dry.*

pie m. *foot.* Se cortó el pie con el vidrio porque no llevaba zapatos. *He cut his foot on the glass because he wasn't wearing shoes.*

piedra f. *stone, calculus.* Tiene piedras en los riñones. *He has kidney stones.* (Syn: cálculo)

piel f. *skin.* El sol puede quemar la piel fácilmente. *The sun can burn skin easily.*

piel amarilla *jaundice.* La hepatitis causa que la piel se ponga amarilla. *Hepatitis causes yellow skin.*

pierna f. *leg.* Un perro le mordió la pierna. *A dog bit him on the leg.*

píldora f. *pill; birth control pill.* Usan la píldora porque no quieren más niños. *They use the pill because they don't want anymore children.* (Syn: pastilla)

píldora para dormir *sleeping pill.* Necesita píldora para dormir porque es nerviosa. *She needs sleeping pills because she is a nervous person.*

pinzas f. pl. *tweezers.* Sacó la espina con pinzas. *She took the sticker out with tweezers.*

piocha f. (coll.) *chin.* El joven tenía una piocha muy larga. *The young man had a very long chin.* (Syn: barba)

piojo m. *head louse.* Tiene piojos porque no se lava el cabello. *He has lice because he doesn't wash his hair.*

pionillo m. (herb) *croton (Croton coresianus). Prepared as a tea and used in treating colic.*

piquete m. *stabbing pain.* Sintió un piquete en el ojo cuando le pegaron. *He felt a stabbing pain in the eye when he was struck.*

placenta f. *placenta.* La placenta es lo que nutre al feto. *The placenta is what nourishes the fetus.*

planta f. *plant.* Ciertas plantas son medicinales. *Certain plants are medicinal.* (Syn: mata)

planta del pie *sole of the foot.* Tiene callos en las plantas de los pies porque anda descalzo. *He has calluses on the soles of his feet because he goes around barefoot.*

pleito m. *squabble.* Tienen pleitos porque no están de acuerdo. *They squabble because they don't agree.*

podrido -a adj. *rotten, decayed, spoiled.* El huevo huele mal porque está podrido. *The egg smells bad because it is rotten.* —v. podrir.

polen m. *pollen.* El polen puede causar alergias. *Pollen can cause allergies.*

polio m. *polio, poliomyelitis.* Los niños deben vacunarse contra el polio. *Children should be vaccinated against polio.*

polvo m. *dust.* Está estornudando porque hay mucho polvo en el aire. *He is sneezing because there is a lot of dust in the air.*

pomada f. *ointment.* Se puede usar pomada en unas quemaduras. *Ointment can be used on some burns.* (Syn: ungüento)

poner en agua *to soak.* Ponga su pie en agua todos los días porque está hinchado. *Soak your foot everyday because it is swollen.* (Syn: remojar)

ponerse *to become or get.* El enfermo se puso mejor (peor). *The sick person became better (worse).*

ponerse chinito *to get goose bumps or flesh.* Al salir de la alberca me puse chinito porque hacía frío. *After getting out of the pool I got goose bumps because it was cold.* (Syn: enchinarse la piel)

ponerse de cuclillas *to squat.* La niña se puso de cuclillas para orinar. *The little girl squatted to urinate.*

ponerse de pie *to stand up.* Póngase de pie, por favor. *Stand up, please.* (Syn: pararse)

ponzoña f. *poison (natural).* Hay unas víboras que tienen ponzoña mortal. *Some snakes have deadly poison.*

por inhalación *by inhalation.* Para destaparse las narices, tomó el medicamento por inhalación. *To unstop his nostrils he took the medication by inhalation.* (Syn: por vapor)

por vapor *by inhalation.* See **por inhalación**.

porquería f. *filth.* Como nunca limpaba su cocina, estaba llena de porquerías. *Since she never cleaned her kitchen it was filthy.*

portar v. *to carry (as a disease).* Los mosquitos portan la encefalitis. *Mosquitos carry encephalitis.*

postema f. *abscess.* La postema en el hueso duró mucho para curarse. *The abscess in the bone took a long time to cure.* (Syns: absceso, apostema)

postemilla f. *abscess (in the mouth).* Le duele la muela porque tiene una postemilla. *Her tooth hurts because she has an abscess.*

pozole m. *hominy stew.* Para hacer pozole cueza la cabeza de puerco con nixtamal. *To make* pozole *cook the head of a pig with hominy.*

preferir v. *to prefer.* Prefiero la pastilla como método para cuidarme. *I prefer the pill as a birth control method.*

preocupado, -a adj. *worried.* Es neurótico porque siempre está preocupado sin saber por qué. *He is neurotic because he is always worried without knowing why.* (Syn: mortificado)

preocuparse v. *to worry.* Nunca me preocupo. *I never worry.*

preservativo m. *condom, prophylactic, rubber.* En la farmacia se compran preservativos para cuidar a la esposa. *Drugstore condoms are bought to prevent pregnancy.* (Syns: condón, hule)

primera regla f. *menarche, first menstrual period.* Tuvo su primera regla cuando tenía catorce años. *She had her first period when she was fourteen.*

probar v. *to taste.* Prueba la medicina, hijo, tiene buen sabor. *Taste the medicine, son, it has a good flavor.*

probar *to test.* El doctor le pegó encima del codo para probar el reflejo. *The doctor taps you above the elbow to test the reflex.*

problema m. *problem.* Hay personas que no pueden soportar los problemas de la vida. *There are people who cannot cope with life's problems.*

procrear v. *procreate.* No puede procrear porque es estéril. *He cannot procreate because he is sterile.* (Syn: engendrar)

profundo, -a adj. *deep.* El cuerno del toro hace una herida profunda. *The horn of the bull makes a deep wound.*

próximo, -a adj. *next, following.* Tiene que regresar a la clínica la próxima semana. *He has to return to the clinic the following week.*

prueba f. *lab test, examination.* Le hicieron una prueba oncológica para ver si tenía cáncer. *They gave him an oncological test to see if he had cancer.* (Syns: análisis, examen)

prueba de la piel *skin test.* La prueba de la piel se usa para averiguar contacto con tuberculosis. *A skin test is used to verify contact with tuberculosis.*

psicológico, -a adj. *psychological.* Ella no habla porque está en mal estado psicológico. *She doesn't speak because she is in a bad mental state.*

pubis m. *privates, pubic region.* Su pubis picaba a causa de la tiña. *His pubic region itched because of the fungus.* (Syns: empeine, verijas)

pudor m. *modesty.* No permitió el examen físico por pudor. *He did not allow the physical examination because of modesty.*

pudrirse v. *to decay, rot, spoil.* Si la carne se deja al aire, se pudre. *If meat is left out it spoils.*

puerco, -a adj. *dirty.* El niño trae puercas las manos. *The child has dirty hands.* (Syn: sucio)

pujido m. *grunt.* Cuando el niño tuvo pulmonía resolló con pujidos. *When the child had pneumonia he grunted when he breathed.*

pujo m. *grunting; desire to evacuate, tenesmus.* Después de la operación tuvo pujo. *After the operation he had tenesmus.*

pujos m. pl. (ethn.) *folk concept that if a newly delivered or menstruating woman touches an infant, she can cause him to strain pathologically.* No es verdad que la mujer durante la regla cause pujo a los niños. *It is not true that a menstruating woman can cause straining in children.*

pulga f. *flea (pulex).* La picada de la pulga da mucha comezón. *The bite of the flea is very itchy.*

pulmón m. *lung.* Los cigarros causan daño a los pulmones. *Cigarettes cause damage to the lungs.*

pulmonía f. *pneumonia.* Su catarro se convirtió en pulmonía porque no se cuidaba. *His cold turned into pneumonia because he didn't take care of himself.*

pulso m. *pulse.* Tocó la muñeca del herido para ver si tenía pulso. *He felt the injured man's wrist to see if he had a pulse.*

puntada f. *stitch, surgical suture.* La cortada era larga y fue necesario cerrarla con puntadas. *The cut was long and it was necessary to close it with stitches.*

punzada f. *stitch, sticking pain.* Corrió demasiado y le pegó una punzada. *She ran too much and got a stitch.*

puño m. *fist.* Por favor haga un puño. *Please make a fist.*

puño m. *handful.* Ponga un puño de la yerba en el agua. *Put a handful of the herb in water.*

purgación f. (old) *gonorrhea, clap.* En Sonora, todavía llaman purgación a la gonorrea. *In Sonora, gonorrhea is still called the purge.* (Syns: gonorrea, chorro)

pus f. (coll.) *pus.* La herida infectada creaba pus. *The infected wound developed pus.*

Q

quebradura f. *break, fracture.* Las quebraduras de los huesos de los viejos se sueldan más lentamente. *Fractures knit more slowly in old people.*

quedarse v. *to stay.* Doctor, ¿hasta cuándo tengo que quedarme en el hospital? *Doctor, how long do I have to stay in the hospital?*

quebrarse v. *to break, fracture.* Se quebró la pierna cuando se cayó en el hielo. *He broke his leg when he fell on the ice.* (Syn: fracturar)

quejarse v. *to complain.* Se quejó de un dolor. *She complained of a pain.*

quemadura f. *burn.* La grasa caliente se incendió y le causó una quemadura. *The hot fat caught fire and gave him a burn.*

quemar v. *to burn.* El café caliente que se derramó le quemó la mano. *The hot coffee burned her hand when it spilled.*

quijada f. *jaw, mandible.* No puede mover la quijada porque tiene tétano. *He can't move his mandible because he has lockjaw.* (Syn: mandíbula)

quiste m. *cyst.* Le operaron el ovario porque tenía un quiste. *They took out the ovary because it contained a cyst.*

quitar v. *to remove, take out.* Tenía cáncer de la garganta; le operaron para quitárselo. *He had throat cancer; they operated to remove it.* (Syn: sacar)

quitarle el pecho al bebé *to wean.* Cuando el bebé echa dientes su madre empieza a quitarle el pecho. *When a baby starts to teethe his mother begins to wean him.* (Syn: destetar)

quitarse la ropa *to undress.* El no quería quitarse la ropa ante la doctora. *He didn't want to undress in front of the woman doctor.* (Syn: desvestirse)

R

rabadilla f. *tailbone, coccyx.* Cuando se fractura la rabadilla se siente dolor al sentarse. *Sitting is painful when one fractures the tailbone.* (Syn: cócciz)

rabia f. *rabies, hydrophobia.* Los perros que tienen rabia echan espuma por la boca. *Rabid dogs foam at the mouth.*

rabia f. (coll.) *anger.* Le dió rabia porque no le hacían caso. *He became angry because no one paid attention to him.* (Syn: coraje)

radiografía f. *x-ray.* La radiografía muestra donde está podrida la muela. *The x-ray shows where the tooth is decayed.* (Syn: rayo equis)

rajado, -a adj. *chapped, cracked.* Tenía los labios rajados a causa del viento. *The wind had given him chapped lips.*

rascar *to scratch.* Quería que me rascaran la espalda. *I wanted to have my back scratched.* (Syns: rasguñar, arañar, aruñar)

rasguñar *to scratch.* El gato me rasguñó. *The cat scratched me.* (Syns: aruñar, arañar, rascar)

rasguño m. *scratch.* Tiene un rasguño en su brazo. *He has a scratch on his arm.*

rasparse v. *to scrape, to "skin."* Se raspó la rodilla cuando se cayó el niño. *The child skinned his knee when he fell.* (Syn: rozar)

rasquera f. *itching sensation.* Tengo rasquera en la cortada. *I have an itching sensation in the cut.* (Syn: comezón)

rasurar v. *to shave.* Antes de operar hay que preparar la piel rasurándola. *Before operating, the skin must be prepared by shaving it.*

rata f. *rat.* Las ratas pueden portar la peste. *Rats can carry bubonic plague.*

ratón m. *mouse.* Los ratones pueden portar leptospirosis con el orín. *Mice can spread leptospirosis with their urine.*

rayo equis *x-ray.* Se usa el rayo equis para averiguar si uno tiene t.b. *X-rays are used to determine whether one has TB.* (Syn: radiografía)

reacción f. *reaction.* Tuvo una reacción positiva. *He had a positive reaction.*

receta f. *prescription (med.); recipe.* Para comprar antibióticos uno necesita una receta del médico. *In order to buy antibiotics one needs a doctor's prescription.*

recetar v. *to prescribe (medicines).* El doctor me recetó cápsulas de penicilina. *The doctor prescribed penicillin capsules for me.*

recto m. *rectum.* A causa de la diarrea, le dolió el recto. *His rectum hurt because of the diarrhea.*

regla f. *menstruation, period.* La regla ocurre normalmente una vez al mes. *Menstruation normally occurs once a month.* (Syns: periodo (m.), menstruación)

reglar v. *to menstruate, to have your period.* Las mujeres reglan normalmente cada 28 diás. *Women generally menstruate every 28 days.* (Syns: estar enferma, menstruar)

reírse v. *laugh.* El enfermo se reía porque tenía miedo. *The sick man laughed because he was afraid.*

relajarse v. *to relax.* Los que están nerviosos no pueden relajarse. *Nervous people can't relax.* (Syn: aflojarse)

remedio m. *remedy.* Si uno está enfermo, hay que buscar remedio. *If one is sick, one has to look for a remedy.*

remedio casero m. *home remedy.* A veces los médicos no creen en los remedios caseros. *Sometimes doctors don't believe in home remedies.*

remojar v. *to soak.* Se debe remojar la mano tres veces al día. *You should soak your hand three times a day.* (Syn: poner en agua)

repetir v. *to belch, burp.* Hay que dejar que los bebés repitan después de darles de mamar. *One must allow babies to burp after nursing.* (Syns: erutar, eructar)

resequedad de la piel *skin dryness. It frequently refers to Arizona white spots or sun spots.* Es buena la loción para prevenir la resequedad de la piel. *Lotion is good for dry skin.*

resfriado m. *common cold.* Cuando cambia la temperatura, mucha gente sufre de resfriados. *When weather temperatures change many people get colds.* (Syn: catarro)

resollar v. *to wheeze.* El niño asmático resuella en la noche. *The asthmatic child wheezes at night.*

respirar v. *to breathe.* Respire profundamente y no suelte el aire. *Breathe deeply and hold your breath.*

respirar con dificultad *shortness of breath, dyspnea.* Cuando uno tiene enfermedad del corazón muchas veces respira con dificultad. *When one has a heart disease one is often short of breath.*

respirar por la boca *to breathe through the mouth.* ¡Respire por la boca, no empuje! *Breathe through your mouth, don't push.*

resultado m. *result.* Los resultados del examen médico mostraron que tenía cáncer. *The results of the medical examination showed that he had cancer.*

reumas f. pl. (also **riumas**) *rheumatism, arthritis.* Reumas es una palabra familiar para artritis. *Rheumatism is a colloquial expression for arthritis.*

reventarse v. *to burst.* Se le reventó el apéndice. *His appendix burst.*

rinconera f. *quack midwife (one who delivers babies or aborts them using dangerous or questionable methods).* La rinconera le provocó un aborto a la soltera. *The quack midwife aborted the baby of the unmarried woman.*

riñón m. *kidney.* Le operaron para quitarle un riñón infectado. *They operated on him to remove an infected kidney.*

ritmo m. *rhythm; rhythm method of birth control.* Muchas mujeres dicen que el ritmo no sirve para evitar el embarazo. *Many women say the rhythm method isn't an effective way to prevent pregnancy.*

rodilla f. *knee.* La pelota de béisbol le lastimó la rodilla. *The baseball hurt his knee.*

romero m. (herb) *rosemary (Rosmarinus officialis).* Prepared as a tea and used to bring on a delayed menstrual period.

roncar v. *to snore.* Uno ronca cuando la lengua le tapa la garganta. *One snores when the tongue blocks the throat.*

ronco -a adj. (estar) *to be hoarse.* El estar ronco continuamente puede ser una señal temprana del cáncer. *Constant hoarseness can be an early warning sign of cancer.*

ronquera f. *hoarseness.* El fumar en exceso causa a veces la ronquera. *Excessive smoking may cause hoarseness.*

roñoso -a adj. *scaly.* La piel seca puede estar roñosa. *Dry skin can be scaly.*

ropa f. *clothing.* Cuando hace frío hay que llevar más ropa. *When it's cold it's necessary to wear more clothing.*

rosa de Castilla f. (herb) *rose (Rosa sp.). Petals prepared as a tea and taken as a mild purge.*

rotura f. *hernia, rupture.* No vale fajar el ombligo del niño para prevenir una rotura. *Binding the navel will not prevent a hernia.* (Syn: hernia)

rozadura f. *scrape; chafing.* La camisa tiesa le causó una rozadura en la nuca. *The stiff shirt caused a chafing on his neck.*

rozar v. *to scrape; to chafe.* Algunas mujeres creen que el coil puede rozar la matriz. *Some women believe that the I.U.D. can scrape the uterus.* (Syn: rasparse)

ruborizarse v. *to blush.* Se ruborizó porque la pregunta le pareció indiscreta. *She blushed because the question seemed indiscreet.* (Syn: enrojecerse)

ruda f. (herb) *rue (Ruta graveolens). Fried in lard and used as drops in treatment of earache.*

ruido m. *noise.* Uno se cansa más pronto si hay mucho ruido en el ambiente. *One tires sooner in a noisy environment.*

ruidos en el oído *noises in the ear.* Las alucinaciones pueden producir ruidos en el oído. *Hallucinations can produce noises in the ear.*

S

saber v. *to taste.* La medicina sabe muy dulce. *The medicine tastes very sweet.*

sabor m. *flavor.* Hoy día los jarabes medicinales para niños tienen un buen sabor. *These days medicinal syrups for children have a good flavor.*

sacar v. *to remove, take out, extract.* Es preciso sacar el apéndice antes que se reviente. *It is essential to remove the appendix before it ruptures.* (Syn: quitar)

sacar aire *to burp (a baby).* Es importante sacarles el aire a los bebés después de que maman. *It is important to burp babies after they nurse.*

sacar leche del pecho *to express milk from the breast.* Se puede sacar leche del pecho con una bomba especial. *Milk may be expressed from the breasts with a special pump.*

salida de los dientes f. *teething.* La salida de los dientes es frecuentemente dolorosa para las criaturas. *Teething is frequently painful to children.* (Syn: dentición)

salir la sangre de la nariz *nosebleed.* El aire muy seco puede ser la causa de que salga sangre de la nariz. *Very dry air can cause a nosebleed.*

salirse v. (coll.) *to withdraw.* Para evitar el embarazo, el hombre puede salirse antes de acabar. *In order to avoid pregnancy the man can withdraw before coming.*

saliva f. *spit, saliva.* La saliva viene de la boca. *Saliva comes from the mouth.*

saltar v. *hop.* Salte en un pie. *Hop on one foot.*

salud f. *health.* El comer demasiado no es bueno para la salud. *Eating too much is not good for one's health.*

saludable adj. *healthy.* Es saludable tener algún ejercicio todos los días. *It is healthy to get some exercise every day.*

sanar v. *euphemism for to give birth, deliver.* Ella va a sanar el mes que viene. *She will give birth next month.* (Syn: dar a luz)

sanarse v. *to get well; to heal.* Me sané de la gripa rápidamente. *I got over the flu quickly.* (Syn: aliviarse)

sangramiento m. *bleeding, hemorrhage.* Sufrió un sangramiento después del parto. *She suffered a hemorrhage after giving birth.* (Syn: hemorragia)

sangrar (also sangrear) *to bleed.* Su dedo sangraba porque se había lastimado con el cuchillo. *His finger was bleeding because he had hurt himself with the knife.*

sangre f. *blood.* Ocurre la anemia si falta hierro en la sangre. *Anemia occurs if the blood lacks iron.*

sangre débil *anemia, weak blood.* La sangre débil puede causar cansancio. *Weak blood can cause fatigue.* (Syns: anemia, sangre pobre)

sangre en el orín *blood in the urine; hematuria.* La sangre en el orín es un síntoma de cálculos. *Blood in the urine is a symtom of stones.*

sangre pobre *anemia, weak blood.* See **sangre débil.**

sangrededrago m. (herb) *limberbush (Jatropha cardiophylla).* *Prepared as a tea and used to treat anemia.*

sano, -a adj. *healthful.* El aire del campo es muy sano. *Country air is very healthful.*

sano, -a adj. *mentally sound, sane.* La gente sana por lo general es feliz. *Mentally sound people are generally happy.*

sano y salvo *safe and sound.* Aunque le atropelló el carro, salió sano y salvo. *Even though the car hit him he came out safe and sound.*

sarampión m. *measles, rubeola.* Hoy día hay inmunizaciones para prevenir el sarampión. *Today there are immunizations to prevent hard measles.* (Syn: sarampión malo)

sarampión de tres días *German measles, three-day measles, rubella.* Si una mujer embarazada contrae sarampión de tres dias puede dañar al feto. *If a pregnant woman contracts three-day measles, it can harm the fetus.*

sarampión malo *hard measles, rubeola.* See **sarampión.**

sarna f. *mange, scabies.* La sarna es causada por animalitos debajo de la piel. *Scabies is caused by parasites under the skin.*

sarpullido m. (also sampullido) *rash.* Después de tocar la yiedra, le salió sarpullido. *After touching poison ivy, he got a rash.*

sauce m. (herb) *willow (Salix gooddingii).* Prepared as a tea and used to treat fever.

sauco m. (herb) *elderberry flower (Sambus mexicana). Prepared as a tea and used to treat measles and fever.*

secar v. *to dry.* A causa de lavar tantos trastes, se le secaron las manos. *From washing so many dishes, her hands dried out.*

seco, -a adj. *dry.* Si el aire no contiene mucha humedad, está seco. *If air doesn't contain much humidity, it is dry.*

seguido, -a adj. *frequent, continued.* El orinar muy de seguido puede señalar una infección en la vejiga. *Frequent urination may indicate a bladder infection.*

segundo parto *afterbirth, placenta and membranes.* Anteriormente se enterraba el segundo parto. *Formerly the afterbirth was buried.* (Syn: sobreparto)

semana pasada *last week.* Desde la semana pasada no puede ver. *He cannot see since last week.*

semana próxima *next week.* La cita es para la semana próxima. *The appointment is for next week.*

semana que viene *next week.* See **semana próxima.**

semanalmente adv. *once a week, every week, each week, weekly.* Va a comprar comestibles semanalmente. *She goes to buy groceries weekly.* (Syns: cada ocho días, cada semana)

semen m. *semen.* El semen es el flúido que contiene las espermas. *The semen is the fluid that contains the sperm.*

sensación f. *feeling, sensation.* Tuvo una sensación de vértigo porque se levantó demasiado rápido. *He had a feeling of dizziness because he got up too fast.*

sentaderas f. pl. *buttocks.* El padre le pegó al niño en las sentaderas. *The father spanked the child on the buttocks.* (Syn: nalgas)

sentar v. *to seat someone.* La enfermera sentó al hombre para examinarlo. *The nurse sat the man down in order to examine him.*

sentarse v. *to sit down.* Se sentó en la sala de espera del doctor. *He sat down in the doctor's waiting room.*

sentir bascas *to gag, to feel nauseated.* Sentía bascas porque se había mareado. *He felt nauseated because he had become seasick.*

sentirse v. *to feel.* Se siente mal cuando llega la regla. *She feels ill when her period arrives.*

sentirse caluroso, -a *to feel hot.* Después de correr la milla, se sintió muy calurosa. *After running the mile she felt very hot.* (Syn: sentirse sofocado, -a)

sentirse sofocado *to feel hot.* See **sentirse caluroso.**

sentirse solo, -a *to feel lonely.* Se siente solo porque no tiene amigos. *He feels lonely because he has no friends.*

seña f. *sign.* El resollar puede ser una seña de enfisema. *Wheezing can be a sign of emphysema.*

seso m. *brain.* Un golpe fuerte en la cabeza puede dañar el seso. *A hard blow on the head can damage the brain.* (Syn: cerebro)

sietemesino -a n. *premature baby.* El sietemesino estaba en la incubadora. *The premature baby was in the incubator.*

sífilis f. *syphilis.* Los síntomas de la sífilis pueden quedarse ocultos por años. *The symptoms of syphilis can remain hidden for years.* (Syns: mal de la sangre, infección de la sangre)

sífilis congénita *congenital syphilis.* Un bebé nacido de una mujer sifilítica frecuentemente tiene sífilis congénita. *A baby born to a syphilitic woman frequently has congenital syphilis.*

silbar v. *to whistle; wheeze.* Silba cuando habla porque los dientes falsos no le quedan bien. *He whistles when he talks because his false teeth don't fit well.*

simple adj. *euphemism for mentally retarded.* No puede trabajar porque ha sido simple desde nacimiento. *He cannot work because he has been mentally retarded since birth.* (Syns: inocente, atrasado)

síntoma m. *symptom.* La náusea es un síntoma del embarazo. *Nausea is a symptom of pregnancy.*

sinusitis f. *sinusitis.* Hay dolor de cabeza cuando uno tiene sinusitis. *One has a headache when one has sinusitis.*

sobaco m. *armpit, axilla.* El desodorante le irritó el sobaco. *The deodorant irritated his armpit.* (Syn: axila)

sobador, -a n. (ethn.) *folk healer who massages.* La sobadora frota el codo dislocado. *The sobadora rubs the dislocated elbow.*

sobar v. *to massage.* El sobar a uno le ayuda a relajarse. *Massaging someone helps him to relax.*

sobreparto m. *afterbirth, placenta and membranes.* See **segundo parto.**

soldarse v. *to knit (bones).* Los huesos se sueldan rápidamente en la niñez. *Bones knit rapidly in childhood.*

soltura f. *diarrhea, loose bowels.* El turista sufrió soltura porque tomó el agua sin hervirla. *The tourist suffered diarrhea because he drank the water without boiling it.*

sonarse la nariz *blow the nose.* Se suena la nariz mucho porque tiene catarro. *She blows her nose a lot because she has a cold.*

sonda f. *catheter, sound.* Le vamos a poner una sonda para sacarle orín. *We are going to put a catheter in to take some urine out.* (Syns: tripa, drenaje)

soplo m. *murmur (abnormal heart sounds).* Un soplo del corazón puede indicar que hay algo anormal. *A heart murmur can indicate something is abnormal.* (Syn: murmullo)

sordera f. *deafness.* Padece de sordera porque se dañaron los oídos. *He suffers from deafness because his ears were damaged.*

sordo, -a n. *deaf person.* Los sordos no oyen bien. *Deaf people don't hear well.* —adj. sordo.

suciedad f. *dirt.* Si uno no limpia la casa, se acumula mucha suciedad. *If one doesn't clean house a lot of filth accumulates.*

sucio f. *dirty.* La madre bañó al niño porque estaba sucio. *The mother bathed the child because he was dirty.* (Syn: puerco)

sudar v. *to perspire, sweat.* Sudaba mucho porque hacía calor. *He was sweating a lot because it was hot.*

sudores a chorros *copious perspiration (diaphoresis).* La pulmonía puede causar sudores a chorros. *Pneumonia may cause copious perspiration.*

sueño m. *dream.* Mucha gente dice que la indigestión causa malos sueños. *People say that indigestion causes bad dreams.*

suero m. *curative solution.* Se puede curar la deshidratación con inyecciones de suero. *Dehydration can be treated with intravenous solutions.*

sufrir de *to suffer (something).* No puede caminar bien porque sufre de vértigo. *He can't walk well because he suffers dizziness.* (Syn: padecer de)

sugerencia f. *suggestion.* Esa es una buena sugerencia. *That is a good suggestion.*

suicidarse v. *to commit suicide.* Se suicidó porque estaba deprimido. *He committed suicide because he was depressed.*

suicidio m. *suicide.* La iglesia católica condena el suicidio. *The Catholic church condemns suicide.*

supositorio m. *suppository.* Al niño le pusieron un supositorio para que obrara. *They gave the child a suppository so that he would move his bowels.* (Syn: calilla)

supurar v. *to weep.* La herida estaba supurando mucho. *The wound was weeping a great deal.*

sustancia f. *substance, element.* La leche es una sustancia curativa para las úlceras. *Milk is a curative substance for ulcers.*

susto m. *shock, fright, trauma.* El ver el cadáver le dió un susto. *Seeing the cadaver gave him a shock.*

susto m. (ethn.) *fright. Folk belief that fright can cause delayed or immediate physical damage. Diagnosed and cured by suppositories of garlic in a series of three or nine treatments.* (Syn: tripa ida)

T

tabique m. *septum.* El tabique divide las narices. *The septum divides the nostrils.*

talón m. *heel.* Mientras caminaba lastimó su talón. *While walking he hurt his heel.*

tallarse v. *to wring the hands (in anxiety).* Se estaba tallando las manos a causa de nerviosidad. *He was wringing his hands because of nervousness.*

tamaño m. *size.* Es importante que el diafragma sea de tamaño exacto. *It is important for the diaphragm to be the right size.*

tarantas f. pl. *dizziness.* Algunas mujeres se quejan de que la pastilla anticonceptiva les da tarantas. *Some women complain that the contraceptive pill causes dizziness.*

tarde adv. *late.* El enfermo llegó al hospital demasiado tarde. *The sick man arrived at the hospital too late.*

tarde f. *afternoon.* Debe de volver a mi oficina mañana por la tarde. *You must return to my office tomorrow afternoon.*

tartamudear v. *to stutter.* Muchas veces los niños que tartamudean son muy inteligentes. *Often children who stutter are very intelligent.*

té m. *tea.* El té de manzanilla alivia el cólico. *Chamomile tea soothes colic.*

tecato, -a n. (coll.) *user of heroin.* Es tecato: tiene el vicio de usar heroína. *He is a* tecato: *he has the vice of using heroin.*

tejido m. *tissue.* Trajeron la muestra de tejido al laboratorio. *They took the sample of tissue to the laboratory.*

tela adhesiva *adhesive tape.* Se usa tela adhesiva para pegar la gaza a la herida. *Adhesive tape is used to hold gauze on the wound.*

temblar v. *to tremble.* La niña estaba temblando de miedo cuando la encontraron. *The little girl was trembling with fear when they found her.*

temblor m. *tremor.* Se cree que el aire puede causar temblor del ojo. *It is believed that a draft can cause eye tremor.*

temperatura f. *temperature.* La temperatura normal del cuerpo es 37°C. *Normal body temperature is 37° C.*

templado, -a adj. *mild (weather).* El tiempo templado no trae muchos catarros. *Mild weather doesn't bring many colds.*

tenazas f. pl. *forceps.* A veces se usan tenazas para sacar la criatura durante el parto. *Sometimes forceps are used to extract the baby during delivery.* (Syn: hierros)

tener v. *to have.* Tienen cuatro hijos. *They have four children.*

tener celos *to be jealous.* El siempre tener celos es una enfermedad de carácter. *It is a character disorder to be jealous all the time.* (Syn: celoso)

tener ganas *to feel like doing something.* Desde que se enfermó, no tiene ganas de comer. *Since he got sick, he doesn't feel like eating.*

tener hambre *to be hungry.* Después de trabajar tanto tuvo mucha hambre. *After working so hard she was very hungry.*

tener sed *to be thirsty.* Tenía mucha sed pero no le dejaron tomar. *He was very thirsty, but they didn't let him drink.*

tener sueño *to be sleepy.* El tiene sueño todo el tiempo. *He is sleepy all the time.*

tenso -a adj. *tense.* Está muy tenso por no saber qué va a ocurrir. *He is very tense because he doesn't know what is going to happen.*

tentar v. *to touch, feel (also sexually).* Se tienta la frente para saber si hay fiebre. *You touch the forehead to see if there is fever.* (Syn: tocar)

terco -a adj. *persistent.* El niño sufrió de una tos terca que no se le iba. *The child suffered from a persistent cough that wouldn't go away.*

terminar v. *to finish, end.* En cuanto el doctor termine el examen, Ud. puede vestirse. *As soon as the doctor finishes the examination, you can get dressed.*

testículo m. *testicle.* El testículo forma la esperma. *The testicle makes sperm.*

teta f. (coll.) *breast.* La mujer debe de examinarse las tetas cada mes para señales de cáncer. *A woman should examine her breasts each month for signs of cancer.* (Syns: pecho, chichi)

tétano m. *tetanus, locked jaw.* Se puede inmunizar contra el tétano. *One can immunize against tetanus.* (Syn: pasmo seco)

tetera f. *nursing bottle.* El niño podía sostener la tetera a los cinco meses. *The baby could hold his bottle at five months.* (Syns: mamadera, biberón, botella)

tetilla f. *nipple.* Hay que secar las tetillas para evitar grietas. *The nipples must be dried to avoid cracks.* (Syn: pezón)

tibio -a adj. *lukewarm.* Primero, lávese la herida con agua tibia. *First, wash your wound with lukewarm water.*

tieso -a adj. *stiff.* Después de quitarse el yeso, la pierna permaneció tiesa. *After the cast was removed, the leg remained stiff.*

tiña f. *ringworm, tinea.* La tiña da comezón y es causada por hongos. *Ringworm itches and is caused by fungi.*

tirisia f. (ethn.) *separation sorrow. Meaning originates from the idea that jaundice may be caused by the emotion of sorrow.* Cuando la madre fue al hospital, el niño sintió tirisia. *When the mother went to the hospital the child felt separation sorrow.*

tiritar v. *to shiver.* Está tiritando de frío. *She is shivering from cold.*

tiroideo -a adj. *thyroid.* Es preciso tener yodo en la comida para formar la hormona tiroidea. *It is necessary to have iodine in the diet to form thyroid hormone.*

tiroides m. *thyroid.* Tiene el tiroides hinchado. *He has a swollen thyroid.*

tis f. (coll.) *tuberculosis, T.B.* Tis es el nombre familiar para tuberculosis. *Tis is the colloquial term for tuberculosis.* (Syns: tuberculosis, tisis)

tisana f. *(medicinal) tea.* Uno puede comprar hierbas para tisanas. *One can buy herbs for medicinal teas.*

tísico, -a n. *T.B. patient; sickly (in general).* El hombre delgado parecía tísico. *The thin man looked sickly.*

tisis f. *tuberculosis, T.B.* Hoy día la tisis es principalmente enfermedad de la vejez. *Nowadays tuberculosis is mainly a disease of old age.* (Syns: tis, tuberculosis)

tlachichinole m. (herb) *Kohleria deppeana. Prepared in solution and used as a cleansing vaginal douche.*

tobillo m. *ankle.* Cuando se deslizó en el hielo se torció el tobillo. *When he slipped on the ice, he twisted his ankle.*

tocar v. *touch, feel.* Dijo que le dolió cuando le toqué la oreja. *He said it hurt when I touched his ear.* (Syn: tentar)

tomar v. *to drink.* Cuando uno tiene resfriado hay que tomar muchos líquidos. *When one has a cold he must drink lots of liquids.* (Syn: beber)

torcerse v. *to twist, sprain.* Me torcí el pie. *I sprained my foot.* (Syn: falsearse)

torcido, -a adj. *twisted, crooked.* El niño nació con la columna vertebral torcida. *The child was born with a twisted spine.*

torzón m. *abdominal cramp.* Los torzones pueden afectar varios órganos del abdomen. *Cramps can affect different organs of the abdomen.*

tos ferina *whooping cough, pertussis.* Se puede prevenir la tos ferina. *Whooping cough can be prevented.*

toser v. *to cough.* ¡Tosí tanto anoche que no pude dormir! *I coughed so much last night that I couldn't sleep.*

trabajar v. *to work.* Trabaja de carpintero. *He works as a carpenter.*

tragante m. *esophagus.* Se quemó el tragante por beber ácido. *He burned his esophagus by drinking acid.* (Syns: esófago, boca del estomago)

tragar v. *to swallow.* Masca el chicle pero no te la tragues. *Chew the gum but don't swallow it.*

tranquilizador m. *tranquilizer.* Los médicos pueden recetar tranquilizadores para calmar los nervios. *Doctors can prescribe tranquilizers for calming the nerves.* (Syn: calmante)

trastornos m. pl. *disturbances.* Hay trastornos físicos y mentales. *There are physical and mental disturbances.*

tripa f. *catheter.* Le pusieron una tripa para sacar el orín de la vejiga. *They inserted a catheter to take urine out of his bladder.* (Syns: sonda, drenaje)

tripa ida (ethn.) *locked intestine. Belief that fright can lock the intestines.* La tripa ida puede ser motivada por un susto. Tripa ida *can be caused by a fright.* (Syn: susto)

tripas f. pl. *intestines.* La comida picante puede dar torzones en las tripas. *Hot food can cause intestinal cramps.* (Syn: intestinos)

triste adj. *sad.* El estar triste todo el tiempo es enfermedad mental. *To be sad all the time is a mental illness.*

trompa f. *tube, duct.* La trompa es un término elegante para cualquier tipo de tubo. La trompa *is an elegant term for any type of tube or duct.*

trompa de falopio *fallopian tube.* See **tubo falopio**.

tropezarse v. *to trip.* Se tropezó en el borde de la alfombra y se cayó. *He tripped on the edge of the carpet and fell.*

tuberculosis f. *tuberculosis, T.B.* See **tisis**.

tubo m. *tube. Biological: may refer to bronchi, fallopian tubes, urethra, spermatic cord, etc. Mechanical: catheter, sound.* La hediondilla a vapor alivia la inflamación de los tubos. *Creosote steam aleviates inflammation of the tubes.*

tubo de plástico *I.U.D., coil, loop.* Le pusieron el tubo de plástico a mi esposa después del nacimiento del segundo hijo. *My wife had an I.U.D. put in after the birth of the second child.* (Syns: coil, alambrito, aparatito)

tubo falopio *fallopian tube.* El tubo falopio lleva el huevo del ovario hasta la matriz. *The fallopian tube carries the ovum from the ovary to the uterus.* (Syn: trompa de falopio)

tuétano m. *bone marrow.* Los glóbulos sanguineos pueden examinarse en una muestra de tuétano del hueso. *Blood cells can be examined in a sample of bone marrow.* (Syn: médula)

tullido, -a adj. *disabled, crippled.* Es tullido porque volvió de la guerra con solamente una pierna. *He is crippled because he returned from the war with only one leg.*

tumor m. *growth, tumor.* Un tumor en la matriz puede causar una hemorragia. *A tumor in the uterus may cause a hemorrhage.*

U

úlcera f. *ulcer, open sore.* La comida ácida irrita las úlceras en la boca. *Acid food irritates ulcers in the mouth.*

úlcera gástrica *stomach ulcer, gastric ulcer.* Si uno tiene úlcera gástrica no debe tomar comida picante. *With gastric ulcers, one should not eat hot food.*

ungüento m. *ointment.* El ungüento antibiótico es bueno para llagas. *Antibiotic ointment is good for sores.* (Syn: pomada)

uña f. *finger or toenail.* Si no se cortan las uñas de las criaturas se rasguñan. *If babies nails are not cut, they scratch themselves.*

uña enterrada *ingrown toenail.* El podiatro puede curar la uña enterrada. *The podiatrist can cure ingrown toenails.*

uretra f. *urethra.* Se pone la sonda en la uretra para sacar el orín. *A catheter is put in the urethra to withdraw urine.*

urticaria f. *urticaria.* Urticaria es el nombre científico para ronchas con comezón. *Urticaria is the scientific name for itching hives.*

úvula f. *uvula.* La úvula cuelga en la parte posterior de la garganta. *The uvula hangs down in the back of the throat.* (Syn: campanilla)

V

vacuna f. *vaccination, injection, shot, immunization.* Los niños deben tener vacunas contra la viruela negra. *Children should have smallpox vaccinations.* (Syns: inmunización, inyección, chot)

vagina f. *vagina.* Hay, supositorios anticonceptivos que se pueden meter en la vagina. *There are contraceptive suppositories that can be placed in the vagina.*

vapor m. *steam.* La medicina dada por vapor alivia la tos. *Medicine administered by steam alleviates coughing.*

varicela f. *chicken pox, varicela.* Las ampollas de la varicela no brotan todas a la vez. *The blisters of chicken pox do not erupt all at once.* (Syn: viruela loca)

várices f. *varicose veins.* No se receta la pastilla para las mujeres con várices. *The pill is not prescribed for women with varicose veins.* (Syn: venas varicosas)

vejiga f. *bladder.* Si hay presión en la vejiga hay que orinar. *If there is pressure on the bladder, it is necessary to urinate.*

vello m. *body hair; down.* El hombre tenía mucho vello en el cuerpo. *The man had a lot of hair on his body.*

vena f. *vein.* Murió porque perdió tanta sangre por la vena cortada. *He died because he lost so much blood through the severed vein.*

venas varicosas *varicose veins.* See **várices.**

venda f. *bandage.* Le pusieron una venda en la rodilla raspada para mantenerla limpia. *They put a bandage on her skinned knee to keep it clean.*

venda elástica *elastic bandage.* Le pusieron una venda elástica en el tobillo torcido. *They put an elastic bandage on the sprained ankle.*

vendar v. *to bandage.* Vendó la herida para que no se infectara. *He bandaged the wound so that it wouldn't get infected.*

veneno m. *poison in general.* El arsénico es un veneno. *Arsenic is a poison.*

ver v. *to see.* El viejo ve mal porque tiene cataratas. *The old man sees badly because he has cataracts.*

vergüenza f. *shame, embarrassment.* Muchos no discuten las enfermedades venéreas por vergüenza. *Many people don't discuss venereal diseases because they are embarrassed.*

verijas f. pl. *privates, pubic region.* La tiña puede atacar las verijas. *A fungus can attack the pubic region.* (Syn: partes ocultas)

verruga f. *wart.* Las verrugas negras pueden ser graves. *Black warts can be serious.* (Syn: mezquino)

vesícula biliar *gall bladder.* El dolor que viene de una vesícula biliar inflamada es muy fuerte. *The pain from an inflamed gall bladder is very strong.*

vestirse v. *to get dressed.* Se vistió después de bañarse. *She got dressed after taking a bath.*

víbora f. *snake.* La mayoría de las víboras no son venenosas. *Most snakes are not poisonous.* (Syn: culebra)

vicio m. *vice.* El tomar demasiado es un vicio. *Drinking too much is a vice.*

viento m. *expelled gas, flatus.* Uno puede pasar mucho viento si come frijoles. *Eating beans may cause one to pass much gas.* (Syns: aire, pedo, gases)

vientre m. *womb.* Jesucristo fue la fruta del vientre de Santa María. *Jesus Christ was the fruit of Mary's womb.*

viruela negra f. *smallpox.* Hoy día casi no hay viruela. *Nowadays there is almost no smallpox.*

viruela loca *chicken pox, varicela.* La viruela loca es una enfermedad muy contagiosa. *Chicken pox is a very contagious disease.* (Syn: varicela)

visiones f. pl. *hallucinations, visions.* El tomar peyote puede causar visiones. *Taking peyote can cause hallucinations.*

vista f. *vision.* Tiene vista normal. *He has normal vision.*

vista doble *double vision.* Algunos tienen vista doble cuando toman mucho. *Some people have double vision when they drink a lot.*

vista nublada *blurred vision.* La medicina ocular causa vista nublada por unos minutos. *Eye medicine causes blurred vision for a few minutes.*

viuda negra f. *black widow (Latrodectus mactans).* La picada de la viuda negra es venenosa. *The sting of the black widow is poisonous.*

vivir v. *to live.* Quiero vivir donde no hay humo. *I want to live where there is no smog.*

voltearse v. *to turn over.* Por favor, voltéese para que le examine el otro lado. *Please turn over so that I can examine your other side.*

vomitar v. *to vomit, throw up.* Hay que vomitar algunos venenos. *Some poisons must be vomited.*

vómito m. *vomit, vomitus.* La camisa está manchada de vómito. *The shirt is stained with vomit.* (Syn: basca)

Y

yedra venenosa *poison ivy.* La yedra venenosa puede causar sarpullido en los brazos. *Poison ivy can cause a rash on the arms.*

yema del dedo *finger tip.* Voy a picarle la yema del dedo para sacar una muestra de sangre. *I'm going to stick your finger tip to get a sample of blood.*

yerba f. (var. of **hierba**) *herb.* Uno puede comprar yerbas en la botica. *One may buy herbs in the drugstore.*

yerba buena (herb) *mint (Mentha piperita). Prepared as a tea and used as a treatment for colic.*

yeso m. *plaster (caste).* Cuando mi hijo se quebró el brazo le pusieron un yeso. *When my son broke his arm they put a cast on it.*

Z

zacate m. *grass; hay.* El zacate puede causar jey fiver. *Grass can cause hay fever.*

zancudo m. *mosquito.* El zancudo puede portar el paludismo. *The mosquito can carry malaria.* (Syn: mosquito)

zapeta f. *diaper.* El niño lloraba porque tenía la zapeta mojada. *The baby cried because he had wet diapers.* (Syn: pañal)

zumbidos (del oído) *buzzing noises (in the ear) tinnitus.* Demasiada aspirina puede causar zumbidos del oído. *Too much aspirin can cause buzzing in the ear.*

English to Spanish

ENGLISH
TO
SPANISH

---

abdomen *n.* abdomen m., estómago m.

abdominal cramps cólico m.

abnormal *adj.* anormal.

abortion *n.* *induced abortion* aborto provocado.

abrasion *n.* rozadura f.

abscess *n.* absceso m., apostema f., postema f.

abscess in the mouth postemilla f.

ache *n.* dolencia f., dolor de . . .

ache *v.* doler.

Adam's apple *thyroid cartilage* nuez de Adán, nuez de la garganta.

adhesive tape tela adhesiva.

affect *v.* afectar.

afterbirth *n.* *placenta and membranes* sobreparto m., segundo parto.

afternoon *n.* tarde f.

afterpains *n. pl.* entuertos m. pl.

against *prep.* contra.

aggressive *adj.* agresivo.

agitated *adj.* agitado.

agree with one caer bien.

ailment *n.* enfermedad benigna.

air *n.* aire m.

alcohol *n.* alcohol m.

alcoholism *n.* alcoholismo m.

alleviate *tr.* aliviar.

amnesia *n.* amnesia f.

amniotic sac bolsa de aguas.

amoeba *n.* ameba f., amiba f.

analgesic *n.* medicina para dolor.

analysis of . . . *(blood, urine, etc.)* análisis de . . . (sangre f., orín m., etc.).

anemia *n.* anemia f., sangre débil, sangre pobre.

anger *n.* coraje m., rabia f. (coll.).

angioma *n.* cabecita de vena.

anguish *n.* *(physical)* congoja f.

anguish *n.* *(mental)* angustia f.

ankle *n.* tobillo m.

antiphlogistic *n.* antiflogístico m.

anxiety *n.* ansiedad f., ansias f. pl.

anxiety attack crisis nerviosa

anxious *adj.* ansioso.

appendicitis *n.* apendicitis f.

appendix *n.* apendis m. (coll. var. of apéndice).

appetite *n.* apetito m., ganas de comer.

appointment *n.* cita f.

Arizona white spots resequedad de la piel.

arm *n.* brazo m.

armpit *n.* *axilla* sobaco m., axila f.

artery *n.* arteria f.

arthritis *n.* artritis f.

ashamed (to be) avergonzarse v.

attack *n.* ataque m., acceso m.

axilla *n.* sobaco m., axila f.

B

baby *n.* criatura f., bebé m., "baby" m.
back *n.* espalda f.
bad mood (in a) de mal humor.
bag of waters *amnionic cavity* bolsa de aguas.
balance *n.* equilibrio m., balance m.
bald *adj.* calvo.
ball *n.* bola f.
bandage *n.* venda f.
bandage *v.* vendar.
barefoot *adj.* descalzo.
bathroom *n.* baño m.
beard *n.* barba f., piocha f.
beat *v. (physically)* pegar.
beat *v. (of heart)* palpitar, latir.
bedbug *n.* chinche f.
bedpan bacín m.
bee *n.* abeja f.
beget *v.* engendrar, procrear.
belch *v.* eructar, erutar, repetir.
belly *n.* abdomen m., panza f.
bellyband fajita f.
bend *v.* doblar v.
bend over *v.* empinarse.
beneficial (to be) hacer provecho.
beserk (to go) andar volando.
bewitchment *n.* hechicería f.
bile *n.* bilis f.
biliary stones piedras en el vesículo.
binder *n.* faja f.
biopsy *n.* biopsia f.
birth *n.* nacimiento m.
birth control pill pastilla f., píldora f.

birthmark *n.* lunar m.

bite *v.* morder, picar.

bite *n.* mordida f., picadura f.

blackhead *comedon* espinilla f.

black widow *n.* viuda negra f.

bladder *n.* vejiga f.

bleed *v.* sangrar v., sangrear v.

bleeding *n.* sangramiento m., hemorragia f.

blindness *n.* ceguera f.

blink *v.* parpadear.

blister *n.* ampolla f.

blood *n.* sangre f.

blood clot *thrombus* coágulo m., cuajarón m., cuajo m.

blood in the urine sangre en el orín.

blood relative carnal m. & f.

blood test *hematology* análisis de la sangre.

blow *n.* golpe m.

blow the nose sonar la nariz.

blue *adj.* azul.

blurred vision vista nublada.

blush *v.* enrojecerse, ruborizarse.

body *n.* cuerpo m.

body part parte del cuerpo.

boil *v.* hervir.

boil *n.* *furuncle* grano enterrado.

bone *n.* hueso m.

bone *n.* *(fish)* espina f.

bone marrow medula del hueso tuétano m.

born *v.* nacer.

bottle *n.* botella f.

bowel movement *feces* excremento m., caca f. (coll.).

brain *n.* cerebro m., seso m.

break *n.* quebradura f.
break *v.* quebrarse, fracturar.
break out *v.* brotar n.
breast *n.* pecho m., teta f., seno m.
breastbone *sternum* hueso del pecho, esternón m.
breast-feed *v.* dar de pecho, criar con pecho, dar de mamar.
breath *n.* aliento m.
breathe *v.* respirar.
to breathe *(through the mouth)* respirar (por la boca).
bronchitis *n.* bronquitis f.
bruise *n. contusion* moretón m., magulladura f.
brush *n.* cepilla f.
brush the teeth lavarse la boca.
bullet *n.* bala f.
bullet wound balazo m.
bump *n.* chichón m.
bump *v.* darse en (el) . . .
bunion *n.* juanete m.
burn *n.* quemadura f.
burn *v.* arder, quemar.
burning sensation ardor m.
burning on urination ardor al orinar.
burp *v.* eructar, erutar, repetir.
burp a baby sacar aire.
burst *v.* reventarse.
buttocks *n.* nalgas f. pl., sentaderas f. pl.
buzzing noises zumbidos del oído.

C

cactus sticker espina f., alguate m.
caked breast pezón enlechado.
calculus *n.* piedra f., cálculo m.
callus *n.* callo m.
capsule cápsula f.
cardiac disease enfermedad cardiaca.
carry *v.* portar.
cast *n.* yeso m.
cataract *n.* catarata f., nube del ojo.
catch *v.* agarrar, pegarle a uno.
catheter sonda f., tripa f., drenaje m.
cause *v.* causar.
centipede *n.* ciempiés m.
cerebral vascular accident embolio m., estroc m., derrame del cerebro.
cerebrum *n.* cerebro m.
cerumen *n.* cera f.
cervix *n.* cuello de la matriz.
chafe *v.* rozar.
chafing *n.* rozadura.
change *v.* cambiar.
change of life cambio de vida, menopausia.
chapped *adj.* rajado.
character disorder enfermedad del carácter, enfermedad moral.
charge *v.* cobrar.
charlatan *n.* charlatán m., merolico m.
check-up *n.* chequeo general médico.
cheek *n.* cachete m., mejilla f.
chest *thorax* pecho m.
chew *v.* mascar.
chicken pox *varicela* viruela loca, varicela f.

child *n.* chamaco, -a m. & f.; niño, -a m. & f.

childbed fever pasmo del parto.

childbirth *n.* parto m.

chills *n.* escalofríos m. pl.

chin barba f., piocha f.

choke *v.* atragantarse, ahogarse.

cholecystitis *n.* mal de hiel, bilis f., dolor de la vesícula biliar.

chronic disease enfermedad crónica.

clavicle *n.* clavícula f.

clean *v.* limpiar.

cleanliness *n.* aseo m.

clear *adj.* claro.

cleft palate abertura del paladar, boquinete m.

clench *v.* morder (teeth), apretar (fist).

climax *v. (sexually)* acabar.

cling to *v.* pegarse.

clitoris *n.* pepa f. (clitoris).

cloasma *n.* paño m.

close *v.* cerrar.

clothing *n.* ropa f.

coccidiodomycosis *n.* fiebre del valle.

coccyx *n.* colita f., cóccix m.

cockroach *n.* cucaracha f.

coil *n.* coil m., alambrito m., aparatito m., tubo de plástico.

coitus *n.* coito m.

cold *adj.* frío.

cold (common) catarro m., resfriado m.

colic *n.* cólico m.

collar bone *clavicle* clavícula f., hueso del cuello.

collision *n.* choque m.

come to a head madurar.

comedon *n.* espinilla f.

comfort *n.* comodidad f.

comfort *v.* consolar.

comfortable (to be) estar a gusto.

communicable disease enfermedad contagiosa.

complain *v.* quejarse.

complex *n.* complejo m.

complexion *n.* cutis m.

complication *n.* complicación f.

compress *n.* compresa f.

condom condón m., hule m., preservativo m.

congenital disease enfermedad congénita.

congenital hip cadera dislocada de nacimiento.

congenital malformation defecto de nacimiento, deformidad f., deformación congénita.

congenital syphilis sífilis congénita.

congested *adj.* constipado.

congestion of . . . congestión de . . .

console *v.* consolar.

constipated *adj.* estreñido.

constipation *n.* estreñimiento m.

contagious *adj.* contagioso, pegajoso.

content *adj.* contento.

contraceptive *adj.* anticonceptivo.

contraceptive *n.* anticonceptivo.

contraceptive jelly gelatina anticonceptiva.

contractions *n. pl.* dolores del parto.

contusion *n.* contusión f., moretón m., magulladura f.

convenience *n.* comodidad f.
convulsions *n. pl.* convulsiones f. pl.
convulsions resulting from fever alferecía f.
cooked *adj.* cocido.
cooking oil aceite de comer.
cool *adj.* fresco.
corn *n.* callo m.
cotton *n.* algodón m.
cough *v.* toser.
cough up *v.* escupir.
cracked *adj.* rajado.
cramp *n. (abdominal)* torzón m.
crack *fissure* grieta f.
crab louse ladilla f.
cramp *n. (muscular)* calambre m.
cranium *n.* cráneo m.
craving *n.* antojo m.
crawl *v.* gatear.
craziness *n.* locura f.
crazy *adj.* loco.
crib *n.* cuna f.
crippled *adj.* cojo, tullido.
crooked *adj.* torcido.
cross-eyed *adj.* bizco.
crown *n.* corona f., coronilla f.
crush *v.* machucar.
crutch *n.* muleta f.
cry *v.* llorar.
curative solution suero m.
custom *n.* costumbre f.
cut *n. laceration* cortada f.
cut *v.* cortar.
cyst *n.* quiste m.

D

damage *v.* hacer daño.

damp *adj.* húmedo.

dandruff *n.* caspa f.

dangerous *adj.* peligroso.

dead *adj.* muerto.

deaf *adj.* sordo.

deafness *n.* sordera f.

death *n.* muerte f.

decay *v.* pudrir.

decayed tooth or molar muela podrida.

deep *adj.* profundo.

deficiency *n.* carencia f., deficiencia f.

dehydrate *v.* deshidratar.

delirium *n.* desvarío m., delirio m.

deliver *v.* ayudar o asistir al parto.

delivery *n. parturition* parto m.

denture *n.* dentadura f.

develop *v.* desarrollarse.

diabetes *n.* diabetes f. (var. diabetis), azúcar en el orín.

diaper *n.* zapeta f. pañal m.

diaphoresis *n.* sudores a chorros m. pl.

diaphragm *n.* diafragma m.

diarrhea *n.* diarrea f., soltura f., excremento suelto.

die *v.* morir, fallecer.

diet *n.* dieta f.

difficulty *n.* dificultad f.

difficulty in . . . dificultad en . . .

digestion *n.* digestión f.

diphtheria *n.* difteria f.

dirt *n.* suciedad f.

dirty *adj.* sucio, puerco (coll.).

disabled *adj.* tullido.

disagree with one caerse mal.

discharge *n.* desecho m.

discomfort molestia f.

disease of ... enfermedad de ..., mal de ...

disease of social pathology enfermedad de carácter, enfermedad moral.

disgust *n.* asco m.

dislocation *n.* dislocación f.

displacement *n.* descompostura f.

distracted (to be) andar volado (coll.).

disturbance *n.* *(mental)* trastorno m. (mental).

dizziness tarantas.

dizzy (to become) atarantarse.

doctor *n.* doctor, m. & f.; médico, -a m. & f.

double vision vista doble.

douche lavado vaginal.

drain *n.* drenaje m.

dream *m.* sueño m.

dress *v.* vestirse.

drink *v.* tomar, beber.

drip *v.* gotear.

drool *v.* babear.

drop *n.* gota f.

drown *v.* ahogarse.

drowsy *adj.* amodorrado.

drug *n.* droga f.

drug addict drogadicto.

drugstore botica f., farmacia f.

drunk *adj.* borracho.

drunk (to get) emborracharse.

dry *adj.* seco.

dry *v.* secar.

dryness of the skin resequedad de la piel.

dust *n.* polvo m.

dysentery *n.* disentería f., obrar con sangre.
dyspepsia *n.* dispepsia f., estómago sucio indigestión f.
dysphagia *n.* dificultad al tragar.
dyspnea *n.* dificultad al respirar.
dyspneic *adj.* corto de réspiración.
dysuria *n.* dolor al orinar.

E

each week cada ocho días, cada semana, semanalmente.
ear *n. (external)* oreja f.
ear *n. (middle and inner)* oído m.
earache *n.* dolor de oído.
egg *n.* huevo m., óvulo m.
egg white claro m.
elastic bandage venda elástica.
elbow *n.* codo m.
element *n.* sustancia f.
embarrassed (to be) avergonzarse v.
emotion *n.* emoción f.
encourage *v.* animar.
end *v.* acabar, terminar.
enema *n.* lavativa f., enema f.
engender *v.* engendrar, procrear.
engorged nipple pezón enlechado.
enlarged heart corazón grande.
entrails *n. pl.* entrañas f. pl.
envy *n.* envidia f.
epidemic *n.* epidemia f.
epigastrium *n.* boca del estómago.
epilepsy *n.* epilepsia f.

equilibrium *n.* equilibrio m., balance m.
eruption of the skin sarpullido, sampullido.
eruption of the teeth dentición f., la salida de los dientes.
erysipelas *n.* erisipela, dicipela (rare).
esophagus *n.* esófago m., boca del estómago tragante m.
evaporated milk leche evaporada, leche de bote.
every week cada ocho días, cada semana, semanalmente.
evil eye mal ojo.
examination *n.* examinación f.
excrement *n.* excremento m.
exhausted *adj.* agotado.
expecting (to be) estar con familia.
express milk from the breast sacar leche del pecho.
extract *v.* sacar, quitar.
eye *n.* ojo m.
eye dropper gotero m.
eye gnat *hippelates* bobito m.
eyebrow *n.* ceja f.
eyelash *n.* pestaña f.
eyelid *n.* párpado m.

F

face *n.* cara f.
face down boca abajo.
face up boca arriba.
fail *v.* fallar, fracasar
faint *v.* desmayarse.

fall down *v.* caerse.

fallopian tube trompa de falopio, tubo falopio.

falsehood *n.* mentira f.

fart *n.* pedo m.

fast *v.* ayunar.

fast heart beat palpitación f.

fat *adj.* gordo.

fat *n.* gordura f.

fatigue *n.* cansancio m., fatiga f.

fatigued *adj.* agotado.

fear *n.* miedo m.

fearful *adj.* miedoso.

feces *n.* excremento m., caca f., deposición f.

feel *v.* *(emotionally)* sentir(se).

feel *v.* *(manually)* tocar, tentar.

feel (like doing . . .) tener ganas de . . .

feeling *n.* sensación f.

fetus *n.* feto m.

fever *n.* fiebre f., calentura f.

fight *v.* pelear.

fill *v.* llenar.

filth *n.* porquería f.

filthy *adj.* asqueroso, inmundo.

finger *n.* dedo m.

finger tip yema del dedo.

finish *v.* terminar, acabar.

fissure *n.* grieta f.

fist *n.* puño m.

fits *n.* *pl.* convulsiones f. pl.

fix *v.* arreglar, componer.

flank pain mal de ijar.

flatus *n.* pedo m., viento m., aire m.

flavor *n.* sabor m.

flea *n. pulex* pulga f.
flesh *n.* carne f.
flow *v. (menstrual)* bajar la regla.
flu *n.* gripe f., gripa f.
fly *n. musca* mosca f.
foam *n.* espuma f.
focus *v.* enfocar la vista.
fontanel *n.* mollera f.
foot *n.* pie m.
forceps *n. pl.* hierros m. pl., tenazas f. pl.
forehead *n.* frente f.
fracture *n.* quebradura f.
fracture *v.* quebrarse, fracturar.
free *adj.* gratis.
fresh *adj.* fresco.
fresh milk leche fresca, leche de vaca.
fright *n.* susto m.
frightened (to become) asustarse v.
frigidity *n.* frío en la matriz.
from the waist down de la cintura para abajo.
from the waist up de la cintura para arriba.
fungi *n. pl.* hongos m. pl.
furuncle *n.* grano enterrado.

G

gag *v.* sentir bascas.
gall bladder vesícula biliar.
gall bladder disease *cholecystitis* dolor de la vesícula biliar, mal de hiel, bilis f.
gangrene *n.* gangrena f.
gargle gárgaras (hacer).

gas *n. flatus* viento m., aire m., pedo m., gas m.

gastric ulcer úlcera gástrica.

gauze *n.* gasa f.

genitals partes ocultas, verijas f. pl.

germ *n.* microbio m.

German measles *rubella* sarampión de tres días.

get angry enojarse.

get better *v.* mejorarse.

get chills entrar calores.

get dressed vestirse.

get larger hacerse más grande, engrandecerse v.

get smaller disminuirse.

get sick enfermarse.

get up levantarse.

get used to acostumbrarse.

get well sanarse, aliviarse.

get worse agravarse, empeorarse.

girdle *n.* faja f.

girl *n.* chamaca f., muchacha f., niña f.

give birth sanar v., dar a luz.

give out *v.* fallar.

glairy *adj.* claro.

gland *n.* glándula f.

go beserk andar volado (coll.).

go to the bathroom ir al baño.

goiter *n.* bocio m., buche m.

gonorrhea *n.* gonorrea f., purgación f., chorro m.

good *adj.* bueno.

goose bumps (to get) enchinarse la piel, ponerse chinito.

gout *n.* gota f.

grab *v.* agarrar.
grass zacate m.
grippe gripe f., gripa f.
groin *n.* aldilla f., ingle f.
grow *v.* crecer.
growth *tumor* tumor m.
grunt *n.* pujido m.
gullet *n.* boca del estómago, esófago m.
gum *n.* encía f.
gush *n.* *(of fluid)* chorro m.
guts *n. pl.* entrañas f. pl.
gynecologist *n.* ginecólogo, -a m. & f.

H

hair *n.* pelo m., cabello m. (of head), vello m. (of body, especially pubic hair).
half *n.* mitad f.
hallucinations *n. pl.* alucinaciones f. pl., visiones f. pl.
hand *n.* mano f.
handful *n.* puño m.
hangover *n.* cruda f.
hangover (to have) estar crudo.
Hansen's disease lepra f.
happy *adj.* feliz, alegre.
hard *adj.* duro.
hard measles *rubeola* sarampión malo.
hare lip labio cucho, labio leporino.
harm *v.* dañar.
harmful *adj.* dañoso.
have *v.* tener.
hay fever jey fiver, fiebre del heno.

head *n.* cabeza f.
headache *n.* dolor de cabeza.
heal *v.* sanarse.
health *n.* salud f.
health department centro de salud.
healthful *adj.* sano.
healthy *adj.* saludable.
hear *v.* oír.
heart *n.* corazón m.
heart attack ataque al corazón, infarto.
heart disease mal del corazón.
heartbeat *n.* latido m., lato m.
heartbeat (rapid) palpitación f.
heartburn *n.* acedías f., acidez f., agruras del estómago.
heat *n.* calor m.
heavy *adj.* pesado.
heel *n.* talón m.
hematology *n.* análisis de la sangre.
hematuria *n.* sangre en el orín.
hemorrhage *n.* hemorragia f., sangramiento m.
hemorrhoids *n. pl.* almorranas f. pl.
hepatitis *n.* hepatitis f.
herb *n.* hierba f., yerba f.
hereditary disease enfermedad hereditaria, herencia f.
hernia *n.* hernia f., rotura f.
heroine user tecato, -a m. & f.
hiccups *n.* hipo m.
hide *v.* esconderse.
high blood pressure alta presión.
hip *n.* *pelvis* cadera, cuadril (coll.).
hit *v.* pegar, golpear.

hives attack *urticaria* sarpullido m., sampullido m.

hoarse (to be) (estar) ronco.

hoarseness *n.* ronquera f.

hole *meatus* hoyito m.

home remedy remedio casero.

hop *v.* saltar.

hordeolum grano en el ojo, perilla en el ojo, orzuelo m.

hormone *n.* hormona f.

hot *adj.* caliente.

hot (to feel) sentirse caluroso, sentirse sofocado.

hot flashes calores m. pl., calofríos m. pl.

hump *n.* joroba f., joma f., giba f.

hunchbacked *adj.* jorobado.

hunger *n.* hambre f. (el).

hungry (to be) tener hambre.

hurt *n.* herida f., lastimadura f., coco m. (coll.).

hurt *v.* doler.

hurt oneself lastimarse, hacerse daño, golpearse.

hydrocephalus agua en los sesos.

hydrophobia *n.* rabia f.

hygiene *n.* higiene f.

hypertension *n.* alta presión arterial.

hysteria *n.* histeria f.

I

idiocy *n.* inocencia f.
illness *n.* enfermedad f., dolor de . . .
immunization *n.* inmunización f., inyección f., vacuna f., chot m.
impact *n.* choque m.
improve *v.* mejorarse.
incision *n.* cortada f.
indigestion *n.* dispepsia f., estómago sucio, indigestión f.
indisposition *n.* malestar m.
induration endurecimiento m., bolita f.
infection *n.* infección f.
inflammation *n.* inflamación f.
influenza *n.* influenza f., gripe f.
ingrown toenail uña enterrada.
inguinal region ingle m., aldilla f.
inhalation (by) (por) inhalación, (por) vapor.
inherited disease enfermedad hereditaria, herencia f.
inhibited *adj.* cohibido.
injection inyección f., chot m.
injure *v.* lastimar, hacer daño.
injure oneself hacerse daño, lastimarse.
injurious *adj.* dañoso.
injury *n.* lastimadura f., herida f., coco m. (coll.).
inseminate *v.* engendrar.
inside *prep.* dentro de.
instep *n.* empeine m.
intercourse (to have) juntarse.
intestines *n. pl.* intestinos m. pl., tripas f. pl.
invalid *n.* inválido, -a m. & f.

itch *v.* picar.
itching sensation comezón f., rasquera f.
I.U.D. *intra uterine device* coil m., tubo de
plástico, alambrito m., aparatito m.

J

jaw *n.* mandíbula f., quijada f.
jealous *adj.* celoso.
joint *n.* articulación f., coyuntura f.
junk *n.* cochinada f.
jaundice *n.* piel amarilla.

K

kid *n.* chamaco, -a m. & f.
kidney *n.* riñón m.
kidney disease mal de riñón.
kleptomaniac *n.* cleptómano, -a m. & f.
knee *n.* rodilla f.
knee cap *patella* hueso de la rodilla.
kneel *v.* hincarse.
knit *v.* *(bone)* soldarse.
knot *n.* nudo m.
knuckle *n.* nudillo m.

L

laboratory test análisis m., prueba f., examen m.

labor pains *contractions* dolores del parto.

laceration *n.* cortada f.

lack *n.* carencia f., deficiencia f.

lame *adj.* cojo.

lard *n.* manteca f.

larynx *n.* laringe f.

last week la semana pasada.

late *adj.* atrasado.

late *adv.* tarde.

laugh *v.* reírse.

laxative *n.* laxante m.

leak *v.* derramar.

left *adj.* izquierdo.

leg *n.* pierna f.

leprosy *n.* lepra f.

lesion of skin grano m.

leukemia *n.* leucemia f.

lick *v.* lamber.

lie *v.* mentir.

lie down *v.* acostarse.

lift *v.* levantar.

light *adj.* ligero, leve.

like *v.* gustarle a uno.

limp *v.* cojear.

lining *n.* forro m.

lip *n.* labio m.

liquid *adj.* líquido.

liquid *n.* líquido.

listen *v.* escuchar.

live *v.* vivir.

liver *n.* hígado m.

local infection herida infectada le cayó pasmo.

lochia *n.* desecho m., flujo m.

lock jaw tétano m., pasmo seco (rare).

lonely (to feel) sentirse solo.

look at *v.* mirar.

loop *n.* alambrito m., coil m., aparatito m., tubo de plástico.

loose bowels excremento suelto, diarrea, soltura.

loosen *v.* aflojar.

lose *v.* perder.

lose weight bajar de peso.

louse *n.* *(head)* piojo m.

lukewarm *adj.* tibio.

lump *n.* bolita f., endurecimiento m.

lump on the head chichón m.

lung *n.* pulmón m.

M

maintain *v.* mantener.

malaise *n.* malestar m.

malaria *n.* malaria f., paludismo m.

mammary gland pecho m., teta f.

mandible *n.* mandíbula f., quijada f.

mange *n.* sarna f.

marrow *n.* médula f., tuétano m.

marry *v.* casarse (con).

mask of pregnancy *cloasma* paño m.

massage *v.* sobar.

masseur *n.* sobador m.

masseuse *n.* sobadora f.

mature *v.* madurar.

measles *rubeola* sarampión, sarampión malo.

meatus *n.* hoyito m.

medicine *n.* medicina f.

medulla *n.* médula del hueso.

membrane *n.* membrana f.

memory *n.* memoria f.

menarche *n.* primera regla.

mend *v.* arreglar, componer, componerse.

meningitis *n.* meningitis f.

menopause cambio de vida, menopausia f.

menstrual discharge desecho m.

menstruate *v.* reglar, menstruar, estar "enferma."

menstruation *n.* regla f, menstruación f., periodo m.

mental *adj.* mental.

mental disease enfermedad mental, enfermedad emocional.

mental disturbance enfermedad mental, trastorno mental.

mental institution manicomio m.

microbe *n.* microbio m.

midwife *n.* partera f. (licensed), comadrona f. (empiric).

migraine *n.* jaqueca f.

mild disorder enfermedad benigna.

mildew *v.* enmohecerse.

milk *n.* leche f.

miscarriage *spontaneous abortion* mal parto, aborto natural.

modesty *n.* pudor m.

molar tooth muela f.

mold *v.* enmohecerse.

mole *nevus* lunar m.

mongolian spot mancha azul.

monstrosity *n.* fenómeno m.

mosquito *n.* zancudo m., mosquito m.

mouse *n.* ratón m.

mouth *n.* boca f.

move the bowels obrar, hacer caca.

movement *n.* movimiento m.

mucous *adj.* mocoso.

mucus *n.* mocosidad f., flema f., moquera f. (coll.).

mumps *n. pl.* paperas f. pl., chanza f.

murmur *n.* murmullo m., soplo m.

muscle *n.* músculo m.

mushy stool caca aguada, excremento aguado.

myocardial infarction ataque al corazón m.

N

nail *n.* uña f.

nausea *n.* náusea f.

nauseated (to feel) sentir bascas.

navel *umbilicus* ombligo m.

neck *n.* pescuezo m., cuello m. (front part), nuca f., cerebro m. (back part).

nerve *n.* nervio m.

nerves *n. pl.* nervios m. pl.

nervous breakdown colapso nervioso.

nevus *n.* lunar m.

next *adj.* próximo.

next week semana que viene, próxima semana f.

nightmare *n.* pesadilla f.
nipple pezón m., tetilla f.
nit *n.* liendre f.
node *n.* nudo m.
noise *n.* ruido m.
nose *n.* nariz f.
nosebleed *n.* salirle sangre de la nariz.
nostrils *n. pl.* narices f. pl.
nourishment *n.* alimentación f.
numb (to be) tener adormecido.
nurse *n.* enfermera f.
nurse *v.* mamar.
nursing bottle mamadera f., biberón m., tetera f., botella f.
nutritious *adj.* nutritivo.

O

obesity *n.* gordura f.
obstruct *v.* atorar, obstruir.
occiput *n.* cerebro m.
odor *n.* olor m.
oil *n.* *(cooking)* aceite de comer.
ointment *n.* pomada f., ungüento m.
once a week cada ocho días, cada semana, semanalmente.
open *v.* abrir.
opthalmologist *n.* oftalmólogo, -a m. & f.
oral vaccine *(sabin)* gotas de polio.
organ *n.* órgano m.
orgasm (to experience) acabar.
orifice *n.* boca f.
outside of fuera de.

ovary *n.* ovario m.
ovuum *n.* huevo m., óvulo m.
oxygen *n.* oxígeno m.

P

pain in . . . dolor de . . .
pain on . . . dolor al . . .
painful urination dolor al orinar.
palate *n.* paladar m.
palm *n.* palma f.
palpate *v.* palpar.
pancreas *n. pl.* páncreas m.
pant *v.* jadear.
paraesthesia *n.* hormigueo m.
paralyzed, to be estar paralizado.
parotitis *n.* paperas f. pl., chanza f.
parturition *n.* parto m.
pass away *v.* morir, fallecer.
patella *n.* hueso de la rodilla.
patent medicine medicina de la farmacia, medicina de la botica.
patient *n.* paciente m. & f.
pee *v.* mear, orinar.
pelvis *n.* cadera f., cuadril m. (animal).
penis *n.* pene m.
perineal care aseo m.
period *n. (menstruation)* regla f., periodo m., menstruación f.
peripheral *adj.* periférico.
persistent *adj.* terco.
perspiration (copious) sudores a chorros.
perspire *v.* sudar.

pertussis *n.* tos ferina.

phallus *n.* falo m.

pharmacy *n.* farmacia f., botica f.

phlegm *n.* flema f., mocosidad f., moquera f. (coll.).

phthirius pubis ladilla f.

physical disease enfermedad física, enfermedad del cuerpo, enfermedad corporal.

physical examination chequeo general, examinación general, examinación completa, examinación física.

pie baldness jiricua f.

piles *n. pl.* almorranas f. pl.

pill *n.* pastilla f., píldora f.

pimple *n.* grano m.

pinkeye *n.* mal de ojo.

pinta *n.* mal de pinto.

pit of the stomach boca del estómago, epigastrio m.

pity (to feel) tener lástima.

place *v.* colocar.

placenta *n.* placenta f.

plant *n.* mata f., planta f.

plaster *n.* parche m., yeso m.

plaster cast yeso m.

play *v.* jugar.

pleased (to be) estar a gusto.

pneumonia *n.* pulmonía f., neumonía f.

point to *v.* indicar.

poison *n.* veneno m., ponzoña f.

poison *v.* envenenar.

poison ivy yedra venenosa.

poliomyelitis *n.* polio m.

polio drops (sabin) gotas de polio.

pollen *n.* polen m.

poor *adj.* malo.

pot-bellied *adj.* panzón.

poultice *n.* parche m.

pour *v.* derramar.

prefer *v.* preferir.

pregnancy *n.* embarazo m.

pregnant *adj.* embarazada, encinta, gorda, con familia.

premature baby sietemesino, -a m. & f.

prenatal care cuidado prenatal.

prescribe *v.* recetar.

prescribe for oneself autorecetarse.

prescription *n.* receta f.

press against *v.* oprimir.

prickling pain hormigueo m.

privates *n. pl.* partes ocultas, verijas f. pl.

problem *n.* problema m.

procreate *v.* procrear, engendrar.

pruritis *n.* comezón f.

psychological *adj.* psicológico.

pterigium *n.* carnosidad del ojo.

pubic region partes ocultas, verijas f. pl.

puerperium *n.* cuarentena f., dieta f.

puff out *v.* hacer buche.

pull *v.* jalar.

pulse *n.* pulso m.

pupil of eye niña del ojo.

purge *n.* purga f.

purple *adj.* morado.

pus *n.* pus f.

push *v.* empujar.

Q

quack *n.* charlatán m., merolico, -a m. & f.
quiet down *v.* callarse.

R

rabies *n. pl.* rabia f.
raise *v. (lift)* levantar.
raise *v. (nurture)* criar.
rash *n.* sarpullido m., sampullido.
rat *n.* rata f.
raw *adj.* crudo.
reaction *n.* reacción f.
realize *v.* darse cuenta de.
rear *v.* criar.
recipe *n.* receta f.
rectum *n.* recto m.
red *adj.* colorado.
redness *n.* enrojecimiento.
reduce *v. (i.e., a fracture)* enderezar.
relax *v.* aflojarse, relajarse.
remedy *n.* remedio m.
remove *v.* sacar, quitar.
rest *n.* descanso m.
rest *v.* descansar.
restless *adj.* inquieto.
restrooms *n. pl.* comodidades f. pl.
result *n.* resultado m.
retarded *adj.* atrasado, simple.
revulsion *n.* asco m.
rheumatic fever fiebre reumática.
rheumatism *n.* reumas f. pl., riumas f. pl.

rhythm method ritmo m.
rib *n.* costilla f.
rib cage costillas f. pl.
right *adj.* derecho.
ringing noises ruidos.
ringworm *n.* tiña f.
rinse *v.* enjuagar.
ripen *v.* madurar.
rock *v.* mecer.
rocking chair mecedora f.
rot *v.* pudrir.
rotten *adj.* podrido.
rough *adj.* escamoso.
rub *v.* frotar.
rubber *n.* hule m., condón m., preservativo
    m.
rubella *n.* sarampión de tres días.
rubeola *n.* sarampión m., sarampión malo.
rump *n.* rabadilla f., nalgas f. pl.
run *v.* correr.
run *v. (the nose)* escurrir las narices.
rupture *n.* rotura f., hernia f.
rupture *v.* rupturar.

S

sad *adj.* triste.
safe and sound sano y salvo.
saliva *n.* saliva f.
sample *n.* muestra f.
sane *adj.* sano.
scab *n.* costra f.

scabies *n.* sarna f.

scalp *n.* casco m.

scaly *adj.* roñoso.

scapula *n.* paleta f., escápula f.

scar *n.* cicatriz f.

scorpion *n.* alacrán m., escorpión m.

scrape *n.* rozadura.

scrape *v.* rozar, rasparse.

scratch *n.* rasguño m.

scratch *v.* rascar, arañar, aruñar, rasguñar.

scrotum *n.* escroto m.

scrub *v. (dishes)* fregar.

scrub *v. (surgical)* lavarse bien las manos.

seasonal sickness condición del tiempo.

seat *v.* sentar.

see *v.* ver.

seizure ataque m., convulsión f.

self-limited disease enfermedad pasajera, enfermedad temporal.

semen *n.* semen m.

sensation *n.* sensación f.

separation anxiety tirisia f.

septum *n.* tabique.

serious disease enfermedad grave.

severe pain dolor recio.

sexual intercourse coito m., acto sexual.

sexual intercourse (to have) juntarse, estar con el esposo/la esposa.

shallow *adj.* leve.

shame *n.* vergüenza f.

sharp pain dolor agudo, dolor clavado.

shave *v.* rasurar.

shed *v. (blood)* derramar.

shiver *v.* tiritar.

shock *n.* susto m., choque m.

shortness of breath *dyspnea* dificicultad al respirar, respirar con dificultad.

shot *n.* chot m., inyección f.

shoulder *n.* hombro m.

shoulder blade *scapula* paleta f., escápula f.

shoulders *n. pl.* espalda f.

sick *adj.* enfermo.

sick person enfermo, -a m. & f.

sickness *n.* enfermedad f.

side *n.* costado m.

sign *n.* seña f.

sinusitis *n.* sinusitis f.

sit down *v.* sentarse.

size *n.* tamaño.

skeleton *n.* esqueleto m.

skin *n.* piel f., cuero m. (coll.).

skin *n.* *(of face)* cutis m.

skin test prueba de la piel.

skinniness *n.* flaqueza f.

skinny *adj.* flaco.

skull *n.* cráneo m.

slap *v.* pegar, cachetar.

sleep *v.* dormir.

sleeping pill píldora para dormir.

sleepy (to be) tener sueño.

sling *n.* honda para el brazo.

sliver *n.* astilla f.

small pox viruela f.

smarting pain escozor m.

smell *v.* oler.

smell *n.* olor m.

smog *n.* humo m.

smoke *n.* humo.

smoke *v.* fumar.

snake *n.* víbora f., culebra f.

sneeze *v.* estornudar.

snore *v.* roncar.

soak *v.* poner en agua, remojar.

soft spot mollera f.

sole of the foot planta del pie.

solution *n.* suero m.

soothe *v.* aliviar.

sorcerer *n.* hechicero, -a m. & f.

sore *n.* llaga f.

sound *n.* sonda f., tripa f., drenaje m.

speak *v.* hablar.

specialist *n.* especialista m.

specimen muestra f.

sperm *n.* esperma f., germen m.

spider *n.* araña f.

spill *v.* derramar.

spine *n.* espina f., columna vertebral, espinazo m.

spit *n.* saliva f.

spit *v.* escupir.

spleen *n.* bazo m.

splint *v.* entabillar.

spoil *v.* pudrir.

spoiled *adj. (food, etc.)* podrido.

spoiled *adj. (child)* chípili, mimado echado a perder.

sponge bath baño de toalla.

spontaneous abortion mal parto, aborto.

spot *n.* mancha f.

sprain *n.* torcedura f., falseo m., dislocación f.

sprain *v.* falsear, torcer.

spread *v.* desparramar, cundir.

sputum *n.* esputo m., gargajo m.

squabble *n.* pleito m.
squat *v.* ponerse de cuclillas.
squatting *adj.* en cuclillas.
squeeze *v.* apretar.
stabbing pain piquete m.
stain *n.* mancha f.
stand up *v.* ponerse de pie, pararse.
starch *n.* almidón m.
stay *v.* quedarse.
steam *n.* vapor m.
stench *n.* hediondez f., hedor m.
sterile *adj.* estéril.
sterility *n.* frío de la matriz, esterilidad f.
sternum *n.* esternón m., hueso del pecho.
stick *v.* pegarse.
sticker *n. (cactus)* alguate m., espina f.
sticky *adj.* pegadizo.
stiff *adj.* tieso.
sting *n. (sensation)* escozor m.
sting *n. (insect)* picada f., picadura f.
sting *v. (insect)* picar.
stink *v.* apestar, heder.
stitch *n. (surgical)* puntada f.
stitch *n. (sticking pain)* punzada f.
stitch in the side dolor de bazo.
stomach *n.* estómago m., abdomen m.
stomach ulcer úlcera gástrica.
stone *n.* piedra f., cálculo m.
stool *n.* excremento m., caca f.
stool with mucus excremento con babas.
straight ahead derecho adv.
straighten *v.* enderezar.
strength *n.* fuerza f.
strike *v.* pegar, golpear.

stroke *n. cerebral vascular accident* embolio m. (lay var. of embolia), estroc m., derrame del cerebro.

strong *adj.* fuerte.

stutter *v.* tartamudear.

sty *n.* grano en el ojo, orzuelo m., perilla en el ojo.

substance *n.* sustancia f.

suck *v.* chupar.

suffer *v.* sufrir, padecer.

suggestion *n.* sugerencia f.

suicide *n.* suicidio n.

suicide (to commit) suicidarse.

sun spots resequedad de la piel.

sunstroke *n.* insolación f.

support *v.* mantener.

suppository *n.* calillo m., supositorio m.

surgeon *n.* cirujano, -a m. & f.

suture *n.* puntada f.

swallow *v.* tragar.

sweat *v.* sudar.

swell *v.* hincharse.

swelling *n.* hinchazón f.

symptom *n.* síntoma m.

syphilis *n.* sífilis f., mal de la sangre, infección de la sangre.

syrup *n. (medicinal)* jarabe m.

systemic weakness achaque m.

T

tablespoonful *n.* cucharada f.

tachycardia *n.* palpitación f.

tail bone *coccyx* rabadilla f., cócciz m.

take advantage of aprovecharse de.

take care of cuidar.

take hold of agarrar.

take out *v.* sacar, quitar.

taste *v.* saber, probar.

tea *n.* té m.

tea *n. (medicinal)* tisana f.

tear *n.* lágrima f.

teaspoonful *n.* cucharadita f.

teethe *v.* echar dientes.

teething *n.* dentición f., salida de los dientes.

temperature *n.* calentura f., temperatura f.

temporary disease enfermedad temporal, enfermedad pasajera.

tenesmus *n.* pujo m.

tense *adj.* tenso.

test *n. (lab)* examen m., prueba f.

test of . . . *(blood, urine)* análisis de . . .

testicles *n. pl.* huevos m. pl., testículos m. pl.

tetanus *n.* tétano m., pasmo seco.

thick *adj.* espeso, -a.

thigh *n.* muslo m., murlo m.

thin *adj.* delgado.

thinness *n.* delgadura f.

thirsty (to be) tener sed.

thought *n.* pensamiento m.

thread *n.* hilo m.

three-day measles *rubella* sarampión de tres días.

throat *n.* garganta f.

thrombus *n.* coágulo m., cuajo m., cuajarón m.

throw up *v.* vomitar.

thumb *n.* dedo gordo.

thyroid *adj.* tiroideo.

thyroid *n.* tiroides m.

thyroid cartilage nuez de Adán, nuez de la garganta.

tick *n.* garrapata f.

tickle *v.* hacer cosquillas.

ticklish (to be) tener cosquillas.

tie the tubes amarrar los tubos.

tight (to be) estar apretado.

tighten *v.* apretar.

tightly *adv.* fuertemente.

tightness *n.* congoja f.

tinea *n.* tiña f.

tingling sensation hormigueo m.

tinnitus *n.* zumbidos del oído.

tired (to get) cansarse.

tiredness cansancio m., fatiga f.

tissue tejido m.

toe *n.* dedo del pie.

toilet *n.* excusado m.

tongue *n.* lengua f.

tonsils *n. pl.* amígdalas f. pl., anginas f. pl.

too much demasiado adj. & adv.

tooth *n.* diente m., muela f.

touch *v.* tocar, tentar.

toy *n.* juguete m.

trachea *n.* tráquea f., gaznate m.

tranquilizer *n.* calmante m., tranquilizador m.

trauma *n.* susto m., choque m.

tremble *v.* temblar.

tremor *n.* temblor m.

trip *v.* tropezar.

tripe soup menudo m.
trouble *n.* dificultad f.
tubal ligation amarrar los tubos.
tube *n.* tubo m., trompa f.
tuberculosis *n.* tuberculosis f., tisis f., tis f.
tuberculous patient tísico, -a m. & f.
tummy panza f., barriga f.
tumor *n.* tumor m.
turn over *v.* voltearse.
tweezers *n. pl.* pinzas f. pl.
twin *n.* cuate, -a m. & f.; gemelo, -a m. & f.
twist *v.* torcerse.
twisted *adj.* torcido.
typhoid fever fiebre tifoidea.

U

ulcer úlcera f., llaga f.
umbilical hernia (to have) desombligado (estar).
umbilicus *n.* ombligo m.
uncomfortable *adj.* incómodo.
undernourished *adj.* desnutrido.
undress *v.* quitarse la ropa, desvestirse.
upset *adj.* agitado.
upset stomach estómago revuelto.
urethra *n.* uretra f.
urinalysis *n.* análisis de los orines, análisis de la orina.
urinary disease mal de orín.
urinary frequency orinar muy de seguido.
urinate *v.* orinar, mear.
urine orina f., orín m.

urticaria urticaria f.
used up, to be acabarse.
uterus *n.* matriz f.
uvula *n.* campanilla f., úvula f.

V

vaccination *n.* vacuna f., inmunización f.,
chot m., inyección f.
vagina *n.* vagina f.
vaginal suppositories óvulos m. pl.
valley fever *coccidiodomycosis* fiebre del
valle.
varicela *n.* viruela loca, varicela f.
varicose veins várices f. pl., venas varicosas.
vein *n.* vena f.
venereal disease enfermedad venérea, enfermedad secreta.
vertebral column espinazo m., columna
vertebral.
vesicle ampolla f.
vision *n.* vista f.
visions *n. pl.* visiones f. pl.
vitiglio *n.* jiricua f.
vomit *v.* vomitar.
vomitus *n.* basca f., vómito m.

W

wailing *n.* llanto m.
waist *n.* cintura f.

walk *v.* andar, caminar.
warm *adj.* templado.
wart *n.* mezquino m., verruga f.
wash *v.* lavar.
wasp *n.* avispa f.
water *n.* agua f. (el).
water on the brain *hydrocephalus* agua en el cerebro.
wax *cerumen* cera f.
weak *adj.* débil.
weak blood sangre débil, sangre pobre, anemia f.
wean *v.* destetar, quitarle el pecho al bebé.
weaning *n.* destete m.
week *n.* semana f.
weekly *adv.* cada ocho días, cada semana, semanalmente.
weep *v.* llorar.
weep *v.* *(skin)* supurar.
weeping *n.* llanto m.
weigh *v.* pesar.
weight *n.* peso m.
wet *v.* mojar.
wheeze *v.* resollar, chiflar, silbar.
whistle *v.* chiflar, silbar.
white *adj.* blanco.
whooping cough *pertussis* tos ferina (term commonly refers to any persistent cough in children).
windpipe gaznate m., tráquea f.
witch *n.* brujo, -a m. & f.
witchcraft *n.* hechicería f.
withdraw *v.* *(sexually)* salirse.
womb *pelvic cavity* vientre.
work *v.* trabajar, obrar.

worm *parasite* gusano m., lombriz f.
worried *adj.* mortificado, preocupado.
worry *v.* preocuparse.
wound *n.* herida f., lastimadura f., coco m.
wring *v.* *(the hands)* tallarse.
wrinkles *n. pl.* arrugas f. pl.
wrist *n.* muñeca f.

X

X-ray *n.* rayo X, radiografía f.

Y

yank *n.* jalón m.
yawn *v.* bostezar.
yellow *adj.* amarillo.

Supplementary
Information

APPENDIXES

FOOD ITEMS

ALIMENTOS m. pl. (food)

MODOS DE PREPARAR
(preparation methods)

asado, -a *roasted*
cocido, -a *boiled, cooked*
de bote *canned*
frito, -a *fried*
guisado, -a *stewed, braised*
helado, -a *frozen*
hervido, -a *boiled*
horneado, -a *baked*

BEBIDAS f. pl.
(beverages)

agua f. *water*
aguardiente m. *brandy, whiskey*
café m. *coffee*
cerveza f. *beer*
cimarrona f. *ice cone*
hielo m. *ice*
jugo m. *juice*

BEBIDAS f. pl. (Cont.)

leche f. *milk*
licor m. *liquor, spirits*
refresco m. *soda pop, any non-alcoholic drink.*
té m. *tea*
tesüino m. *corn beer*
vino m. *wine*

GRASA f.
(fat)

aceite m. *oil*
aceite de cocinar m. *olive oil, cooking oil*
crema f. *cream*
crema de cacahuate f. *peanut butter*
grasa f. *grease, fat*
manteca f. *lard*
mantequilla f. *butter*
margarina f. *margarine*
mayonesa f. *mayonaisse*
yema de huevo f. *egg yolk*

ALMIDÓN m.
(starch)

arroz m. *rice*
atole m. *corn gruel*
avena f. *oatmeal*
bolillo m. *hard white roll*
cereal m. *cereal*
crema de trigo f. *cream of wheat*
fideo m. *vermicelli*
harina f. *flour*
macarrón m. *macaroni, spaghetti*
maizena f. *corn starch*
nixtamal m. *hominy*

pan m. *bread*
pan tostado m. *toast*
tortilla de harina f. *flour (wheat) tortilla*
tortilla de maíz f. *corn tortilla*

POSTRES m. pl.
(dessert)

almendra f. *almond, almond gelatin*
almíbar m. *syrup*
azúcar m. *sugar*
bellota f. *nut, acorn*
bizcocho m. *anise cooky*
chocolate m. *chocolate*
dulce m. *sweet*
galleta f. *cracker, cooky*
gelatina f. *gelatin, jello*
nieve f. *ice cream, ice*
nuez f. *nut, pecan*
paleta (de agua) f. *popsicle*
pastel m. *pie, pastry*
pan dulce m. *sweet roll*
quequi m. *cake*
sorbete m. *sherbet*

VERDURAS f. pl.
(vegetables)

aguacate m. *avocado*
apio m. *celery*
berenjena f. *egg plant*
berro m. *watercress*
calabaza f. *squash*
camote m. *sweet potato*
cebolla f. *onion*
cebolla verde f. *green onion*

VERDURAS f. pl. (Cont.)

coliflor f. *cauliflower*
chícharos m. pl. *peas*
ejotes m. pl. *green beans*
elote m. *corn (on cob)*
espárragos m. *asparagus*
espinacas f. pl. *spinach*
frijoles m. pl. *beans*
garbanzo m. *chick pea*
lechuga f. *lettuce*
legumbre m. *legume, vegetable*
lenteja f. *lentil*
papa f. *potato*
pepino m. *cucumber*
rábano m. *radish*
repollo m. *cabbage*
tomate m. *tomato*
zanahorias f. pl. *carrots*

FRUTAS f. pl.
(fruit)

albaricoque m. *apricot*
cereza f. *cherry*
ciruela f. *plum*
ciruela pasa f. *prune*
dátil m. *date*
durazno m. *peach*
fresa f. *strawberry*
higo m. *fig*
lima f. *lime*
limón m. *lemon*
manzana f. *apple*
melón m. *cantaloupe*
mora f. *blackberry*

naranja f. *orange*
pasa f. *raisin*
pera f. *pear*
piña f. *pineapple*
plátano m. *banana*
sandía f. *watermelon*
toronja f. *grapefruit*
uva f. *grape*

PROTEINA f.
(protein)

biftec m. *steak*
bolonia f. *bologna*
caldo m. *broth*
camarón m. *shrimp*
cangrejo m. *crab*
carne de cordero f. *lamb*
carne de gallina f. *chicken*
carne de puerco f. *pork*
carne de res f. *beef*
carne molida f. *ground beef*
clara de huevo f. *egg white*
cuajada f. *cottage cheese*
chorizo m. *Mexican hot sausage*
hamburguesa f. *hamburger*
huevo m. *egg*
jamón m. *ham*
pavo m. *turkey*
pescado m. *fish*
pollo m. *fryer*
queso m. *cheese*
salchicha f. *sausage*
sopa f. *soup*
tocino m. *bacon*
trucha f. *trout*
yema de huevo f. *egg yolk*

FOOD (alimentos m. pl.)

PREPARATION METHODS
(modos de preparar)

baked horneado, -a
boiled hervido, -a
canned de bote
cooked, boiled cocido, -a
fried frito, -a
frozen helado, -a
stewed, braised guisado, -a

BEVERAGES
(bebidas f. pl.)

beer cerveza f.
brandy, whiskey aguardiente m.
coffee café m.
corn beer tesüino
ice hielo m.
ice cone cimarrona f., raspada f.
juice jugo m.
liquor, spirits licor m.
milk leche f.
soda pop, any non-alcoholic drink refresco m.
tea té m.
water agua m.
wine vino m.

FAT
(grasa f.)

butter mantequilla f.
cream crema f.
egg yolk yema de huevo
grease grasa f.
lard manteca f.
margarine margarina f.
mayonaisse mayonesa f.
oil aceite m.
olive oil, cooking oil aceite de cocinar m.
peanut butter crema de cacahuate f.

STARCH
(almidón m.)

bread pan m.
cereal cereal m.
corn maíz m.
corn starch maízena f.
corn gruel atole m.
corn tortilla tortilla de maíz f.
cream of wheat crema de trigo f.
flour harina f.
hominy nixtamal m.
macaroni macarrón m.
oatmeal avena f.
rice arroz m.
roll (hard white) bolillo m.
toast pan tostado m.

DESSERTS
(postres)

almond, almond gelatin almendra f.
anise cooky bizcocho m.
cake quequi m.
chocolate chocolate m.
cracker, cooky galleta f.
gelatin, jello gelatina f.
ice cream nieve f., helado m.
nut, acorn bellota f.
nut, pecan nuez f.
pie, pastry pastel m.
popsicle paleta de agua f.
sugar azúcar
sweet dulce m.
sweet roll pan dulce m.
syrup almíbar m.

VEGETABLES
(verduras f. pl.)

asparagus espárragos m.
avocado aguacate m.
bean frijol m.
cabbage repollo m.
carrots zanahorias f. pl.
celery apio m.
cauliflower coliflor f.
chick pea garbanzo m.
corn (on cob) elote m.
cucumber pepino m.
egg plant berenjena f.
green beans ejotes m. pl.

green onion cebolla verde f.
legume, vegetable legumbre m.
lentil lenteja f.
onion cebolla f.
potato papa f.
spinach espinacas f. pl.
squash calabaza f.
sweet potato camote m.
peas chícharos m. pl.
tomato tomate m.
radish rábano m.

FRUIT
(frutas f. pl.)

apple manzana f.
apricot albaricoque m.
blackberry mora f.
cantaloupe melón m.
cherry cereza f.
date dátil m.
fig higo m.
grape uva f.
grapefruit toronja f.
lemon limón m.
orange naranja f.
peach durazno m.
pear pera f.
pineapple piña f.
plum ciruela f.
prune ciruela pasa f.
raisin pasa f.
strawberry fresa f.
watermelon sandía f.

PROTEIN
(proteína f.)

bacon tocino m.
bologna bolonia f.
beef carne de res m.
broth caldo m.
cheese queso m.
chicken carne de gallina f.
cottage cheese cuajada f.
crab cangrejo m.
egg huevo m.
egg white clara de huevo f.
egg yolk yema de huevo f.
fish pescado m.
fryer pollo m.
ham jamón m.
hamburger hamburguesa f.
lamb carne de cordero f.
mexican hot sausage chorizo m.
pork carne de puerco f.
sausage salchicha f.
shrimp camarón m.
steak biftec m.
tripe tripa f.
trout trucha f.
turkey pavo m.

APPENDIX B

KINSHIP TERMS

abuela	grandmother
abuelo	grandfather
ahijada	goddaughter
ahijado	godson
bisabuela	great-grandmother
bisabuelo	great-grandfather
bisnieta	great-granddaughter
bisnieto	great-grandson
comadre	co-mother (ritual)
compadre	co-father (ritual)
concuña	spouse's brother's wife
concuño	spouse's sister's husband
cuñada	sister-in-law
cuñado	brother-in-law
entenada	step-daughter
entenado	step-son
esposa	spouse (wife)
esposo	spouse (husband)
hermana	sister
hermano	brother
hija	daughter
hijo	son

madrastra	step-mother
madre	mother
madrina	godmother
marido	husband
media hermana	half-sister
medio hermano	half-brother
nieta	granddaughter
nieto	grandson
nuera	daughter-in-law
padrastro	step-father
padre	father
padrino	godfather
pariente	relative
prima	female cousin
primo	male cousin
sobrina	niece
sobrina política	spouse's niece
sobrino	nephew
sobrino político	spouse's nephew
suegra	mother-in-law
suegro	father-in-law
tatarabuela	great-great-grandmother
tatarabuelo	great-great-grandfather
tataranieta	great-great-granddaughter
tataranieto	great-great-grandson
tía	aunt
tía politíca	aunt-in-law (parent's brother's wife)
tío	uncle
tío politíco	uncle-in-law (parent's sister's husband)
yerno	son-in-law

aunt	tía; tía política (parent's brother's wife)
brother	hermano
brother-in-law	cuñado (spouse's brother); concuño (spouse's sister's husband)
co-father (ritual)	compadre
co-mother (ritual)	comadre
cousin	primo (male); prima (female)
daughter	hija
daughter-in-law	nuera
father	padre
father-in-law	suegro
goddaughter	ahijada
godfather	padrino
godmother	madrina
godson	ahijado
granddaughter	nieta
grandfather	abuelo
grandmother	abuela
grandson	nieto
great-granddaughter	bisnieta
great-grandfather	bisabuelo
great-grandmother	bisabuela
great-grandson	bisnieto
half-brother	medio hermano
half-sister	media hermano
husband	esposo; marido
mother	madre
mother-in-law	suegra

nephew	sobrino; sobrino político (spouse's nephew)
niece	sobrina; sobrina política (spouse's niece)
relative	pariente
sister	hermana
sister-in-law	cuñada (spouse's sister); concuña (spouse's brother's wife)
son	hijo
son-in-law	yerno
step-daughter	entenada
step-father	padrastro
step-mother	madrastra
step-son	entenado
uncle	tío; tío político (parent's sister's husband)
wife	esposa

OTHER USEFUL SOURCES
OF SPANISH MEDICAL TERMINOLOGY

ARRIOLA, DR. JORGE LUIS, ed.

1971   Aspectos de la Medicina Popular En El Area Rural de Guatemala. Guatemala Indígena. Vol. VI, No. 1. marzo.

MARTINEZ, MAXIMINIO

1969   Las Plantas Medicinales de México. Quinta Edición. Ediciones Botas. México, D.F.

PADRON, FRANCISCO

1956   El Médico y El Folklore. Talleres Gráficos de la Editorial Universitaria. San Luis Potosi, México.

RUIZ CORTINES, ADOLFO, et al.

  1931   Sinonimias Populares Mexicanas de
          Las Enfermedades. Publicación de
          Aniversario de la Revista del Bloque
          Nacional   de   Médicos.   Octubre
          1954.

SOBARZO, HORACIO

  1966   Vocabulario   Sonorense.   Editorial
          Porrua S.A. Republica Argentina
          15, México, D.F.

WERNER, DAVID

  1973   Donde No Hay Doctor: Una guía
          para los campesinos que viven lejos
          de los centros médicos. 140 Leland
          Avenue,   Menlo   Park,   California
          94025.

BIBLIOGRAPHY

ROBINSON, DOW F.

    1969   Manual for Bilingual Dictionaries. Vol. I. Summer Institute of Linguistics, Santa Ana, California.

SPICER, EDWARD, ed.

    1977   Ethnic Medicine in the Southwest. University of Arizona Press, Tucson.

TURNER, PAUL and SHIRLEY

    1971   Chontal to Spanish-English Dictionary. University of Arizona Press, Tucson.